Do Sea Salt

The magic of seasoning

Alison, David & Jess Lea-Wilson

Published by
The Do Book Company 2019
Works in Progress Publishing Ltd
thedobook.co

A CIP catalogue record for this book
is available from the British Library

ISBN 978-1-907974-65-6

10 9 8 7 6 5 4 3 2

To find out more about our company,
books and authors, please visit
thedobook.co or follow us **@dobookco**

5% of our proceeds from the sale of
this book is given to The Do Lectures
to help it achieve its aim of making
positive change **thedolectures.com**

Cover designed by James Victore
Book designed and set by Ratiotype

Printed and bound by OZGraf Print
on Munken, an FSC-certified paper

MIX
Paper from
responsible sources
FSC® C163799
www.fsc.org

Disclaimer
The information in this book has been
compiled by way of general guidance
in relation to the specific subject
addressed, but is not a substitute
and not to be relied on for medical,
healthcare or other professional advice
on specific circumstances and in specific
locations. Please consult your GP
before changing, stopping or starting
any medical treatment. So far as the
authors are aware the information is
correct and up to date as at 2019.
The authors and publisher disclaim,
as far as the laws allow, any liability
arising directly or indirectly from the
use, or misuse, of the information
contained in this book.

Contents

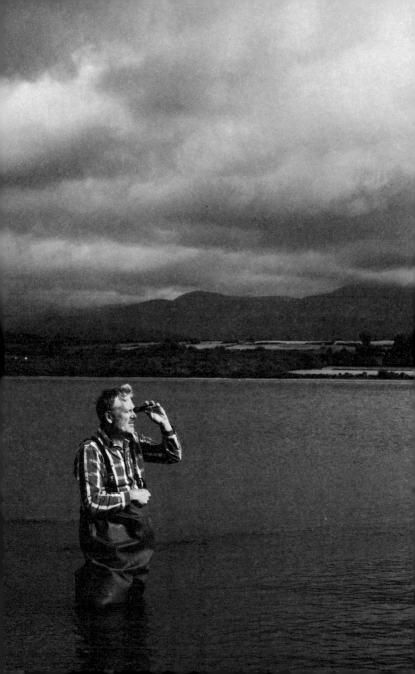

Preface

The cure for anything is salt water:
sweat, tears or the sea

—

Helen Keller

Anglesey, down by the seashore, early morning. The tide is coming in quietly; terns are fishing, having just come back from Africa; oystercatchers are jabbering as they pick up mussels; no one is at work yet. There are no cars on the tiny coastal road; no walkers or birdwatchers. Snowdon is across the Menai Strait — the body of water connecting us to Wales — cloudless, visible and reflected before me. I have work to do on the beach — to check that the seawater is as clean as we say it is before we push the button and start pumping it ashore.

Sometimes I stride in with waders and take a single drop that is then placed on a refractometer. This shows me (by bending light through seawater) how crystal clear the water is and how much sea salt it contains. Sometimes I take my sculling boat and row out until I am over the inlet point to extract a single drop. I need to know that the Gulf Stream has brought us clean salty water, as it has done for the last 22 years, so that we can continue making our sea salt.

This morning was a bit different. Seawater checked, I dispensed with the refractometer and waders before walking to a sandy bit near the slipway for a quick swim. As I swam alone, I started thinking about this book and consciously tried to pin down exactly why the sea has been so important in my life — the foundation of our business, our home and work within walking distance of each other.

Is it the sound of lapping water and sea birds? The smell of seaweed on hot pebbles? Is it the sight of clean water, open skies and deep sand? The touch of cold seawater making your body shrink before a brave dip, giving way to goose pimples and numbness? Putting your head under and having all thoughts suspended for just a few seconds? Perhaps most of all, it's the taste of the sea itself. A single drop licked off your lips after a sea swim tastes of being alive. Yes, this book is about being alive.

It will, we hope, answer many of the questions we are asked about sea salt every day. These questions come from visitors to our ultra-sustainable salt cote building; users of our Halen Môn (Welsh for 'Anglesey Salt') products — from home cooks to world-famous chefs; and curious people from the many food shows we have exhibited at around the world. This is the distillation of our knowledge in a handbook designed to be read, used, shared and put in a pocket or bag — not on the coffee table. I use the word distillation carefully because that's precisely what we do with the seawater, but more of that to come.

—

David Lea-Wilson

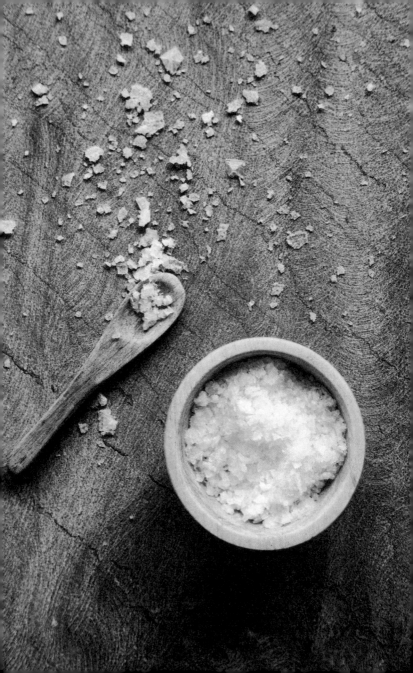

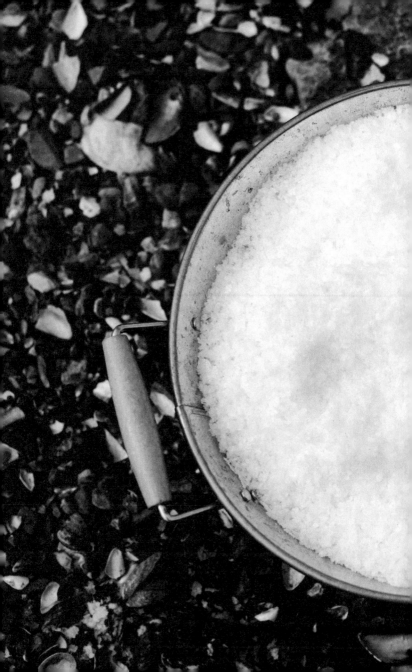

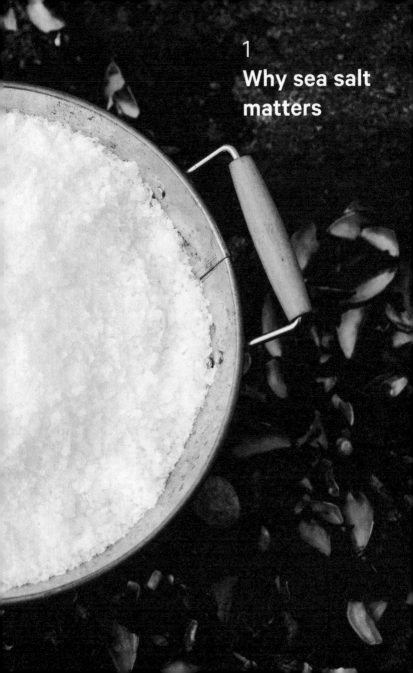

1
Why sea salt matters

*The curled wave is torn carefully
to bring you these crystals*

—

Steve Griffiths, poet

Salt is magical.

Samin Nosrat says that salt is one of the four foundations
of cooking. Anna Jones says ingredients often need
nothing but a scattering of good sea salt to shine; and
Yottam Ottolenghi says salt is 'vital' in any dish, both
sweet and savoury.

What other single ingredient not only enhances our
food to make the other components taste more of
themselves, but brings all the elements of a dish together
so it sings with deliciousness?

Any chef worth their salt knows that it's the most
important ingredient in their kitchen. We often hear that
the ability to season correctly is what separates an average
cook from an outstanding one.

As a humble kitchen staple, salt has an unusual
dimension too — it is physically needed for the human
body to survive. Essential for numerous bodily functions,
the sodium and potassium in salt is so crucial that even
messages to the brain depend upon its presence. The right
electrolytic balance comes from the electrical differences
inside and outside each cell — a bit like having the
correct voltage batteries inserted the right way round in

an appliance. Yet our bodies have no way of storing the electric currents that are partially derived from salts, so we must eat a source of sodium and potassium regularly.

But it's not just about survival. What about our general well-being? Research has shown that people living within one kilometre of the coast are thought to be happier. Victorian Britain loved seaweed and saltwater bathhouses for intense relaxation. Today, we notice that our salt team are pretty healthy and colds are occasional. People are rarely off sick. This could be because making salt is a good job with a great view, but could there also be health benefits to working in a salty atmosphere?

———————

The start of our own obsession with sea salt began in 1997. Back then we had set up and were running an aquarium as a tourist attraction. For nearly 15 years, it showcased the wide variety of sealife to be found around our small but beloved Welsh island of Anglesey. We held a licence from the Queen, who, we had soon found out, owns the coastline of the United Kingdom, so by law we had to pay The Crown Estate for an annual licence to have the right to extract the seawater that we pumped ashore to fill our tanks.

We quickly realised that the raw material which sustained all our sealife — the seawater itself — was exceptionally clean. Much to our surprise, we were able to breed notoriously fussy seahorses, because they were content in their sparkling environment. So when tourism numbers began to drop and times were tough, we began to think about what else we could do with that seawater.

After a lot of brainstorming (and discarding some pretty awful ideas), we made our first batch of sea salt, armed with simple curiosity, a saucepan and an Aga.

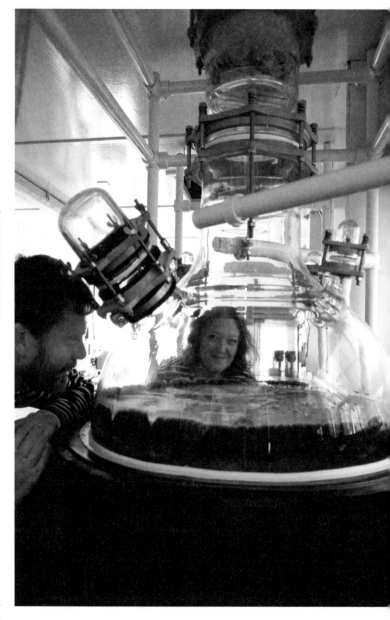

What happened that day was no major breakthrough, but there was enough promise in that pan and process to get us excited. In hindsight, perhaps it was always meant to be. Alison's mother's maiden name is — you guessed it — Salt (they used to live next door to the Peppers too, but that's another story).

Something about starting with a liquid — an overlooked raw material that we were surrounded by — and ending up with a solid element so pure and so *vital*, was magical. There was no doubt about it, we were hooked.

While it's true that anyone can make sea salt (and later in the book, we encourage you to have a go) what we have discovered by making it every day for more than 20 years is that the mastery of the process is both an art and a science. Even now, we are still learning what a vast and complex entity the sea is.

Over the past two decades we have travelled the world over to see how different cultures make salt, both from the sea and the ground. We've been down mines in Krakow and onto stark flats in Trapani, to Guérande for grey salt and to Essex for white salt. We've snuck into countless chemistry classes at our local university (we still do, sometimes, though we usually call ahead now) to learn everything we can. Not to mention the fact that salt has been the gift given to us from every friend's holiday for longer than we care to remember.

Quite apart from sodium chloride (the main component of sea salt), there are *lots* of elements in seawater, and this can be the challenge of making sea salt on a larger scale. When we analysed our Atlantic brine ('brine' is the term commonly used to describe salty water) in chemistry labs, we found that it contained more than 30 different elements, from potassium to magnesium, selenium, zinc and even copper. In fact, much of the periodic table is found in seawater. Eating sea salt means that as well as sodium, you will get a variety of other elements in your salt crystals — many of which are absolutely essential to human health.

Even the seasons make a difference to the make-up of seawater. Seashells, which extract calcium from the water, generally grow much quicker in summer than winter — so you'll find there is more calcium in the seawater in winter than summer.

———

'Salt is so common, so easy to obtain, and so inexpensive that we have forgotten that from the beginning of civilisation until about a century ago salt was one of the most sought-after commodities in human history.'

—

Mark Kurlansky, *Salt: A World History*

So often today, salt is vilified. Being — understandably — concerned about their health, many consumers fear it in any quantity. Perhaps you're one of them. But, to put it bluntly, we have written this book to change your mind: and to tackle the issue of health head on.

Undoubtedly, like most things, too much salt is bad for you. But we want to enthuse you with our love of the ingredient. To look at how different cultures and countries make it. To look at how *you* can make it. To explore seasoning as one of life's essential skills, and to show how this one element has the power to take food from bland to brilliant. In short, we want to treat this humble ingredient with the respect it deserves.

But perhaps in order to look forward, we should look back, because around the world and over the centuries, salt has been highly prized and respected. It has a colourful and important history.

———————

'Let there be work, bread, water and salt for all.'

——

Nelson Mandela

For thousands of years, salt was essential for preserving foods through long winters. Many of the extended voyages made in the era of naval exploration from the fifteenth century onwards depended upon sailing with salted meat contained in barrels. Right up until the twentieth century salt was used to preserve herrings, anchovies and meat as standard practice. And, throughout the centuries, if you weren't near a source, it was almost impossible to produce your own salt, making it an incredibly valuable commodity. Because of this, in most countries, production and import were highly controlled. Remnants of this practice still exist in modern times — in Switzerland for example, the government keeps track of all the salt coming into the country.

A lot of our language reflects the value we used to place on the ingredient. The word 'salary' comes from the Latin *sal*, meaning salt. Historians differ in their interpretation: Roman soldiers were either paid in salt, so were literally 'worth their salt', or were given money to buy it. Either way, the link between value and salt became embedded in our language.

The value of salt in Britain was once so high that it was akin to gold. In the Middle Ages, salt was such a significant commodity that if gold was not available for trade deals, salt was used instead. Salt cellars — containers that held salt on the table — became ornate status symbols and how near to the salt you were seated at important dinners indicated your social standing. If you visit the Tower of London today there is a display of the royal salt cellars, many of which are over 30cm/12in high and made of silver and gold. 'Below the salt' came to mean common or poor. If these people wanted to season their food, they had to be invited to do so. Nowadays, people 'worth their salt' are competent, while those known as 'salt of the earth' — a reference from the Bible — are considered kind and honest.

Salt production and who has control over it has been fought over around the world for centuries. During the period of the British Empire, India made its own salt. But in 1804, Indian salt became a British monopoly and within 10 years, it was illegal for anyone other than the British government to manufacture it. This caused horrific hardship for the Indian people. The British government tried to stop illegal trade, planting an enormous thorn hedge barrier. At its greatest length it ran from the Punjab in the northwest to the state of Orissa, near the Bay of Bengal, in the southeast. It was 14 feet high, 12 feet thick and 2,500 miles long, with a customs post at every mile and 14,000 people managing it.

Famously, Mohandas Gandhi used the campaign against the salt monopoly as a tool to gain independence (the salt *satyagraha*). In 1930 he and a few dozen followers set out to walk 240 miles to the sea where they would break British law and harvest their own salt. After 25 days of marching Gandhi reached the sea. Instead of the 78 people he had left with, he now had thousands behind him. He gathered some salt and changed Indian history forever.

In 1931, it was agreed that Indian people should be allowed to collect their own salt. Lord Irvin, Viceroy of India, suggested they drink a cup of tea together to seal the pact. Gandhi said his drink would be 'water, lemon and a pinch of salt'.

As well as being prized for its financial value, salt was highly symbolic. During ancient times, agreements and weddings in the Middle East were sealed by a salt agreement. A person from each party would take a pinch of salt from their pouch and place it in the pouch of the other. This agreement could not be broken unless an individual could retrieve their own grains of salt.

Closer to home, a Welsh custom from the Middle Ages was that when someone died, a plate containing bread and salt was placed on top of the deceased's coffin. A local 'sin eater' — the poor soul — would then arrive. Their job would be to consume the offerings, supposedly along with sins of the dearly departed, ensuring their swift ascent to heaven.

While we're not suggesting a return to some of these darker traditions from the Middle Ages, we do think salt deserves a little more respect than we bestow on it nowadays. For a seemingly ordinary ingredient, it has undeniably shaped history and is rich with symbolism. Chefs know the value of proper seasoning. But in general culture, we only seem to discuss salt in the context of over-processed food and heart disease (more on that later).

One country with a suitable reverence for salt today is Japan. Back in the 1990s, our travels and research meant we tried dozens of different ways of making salt, but it wasn't until we found a museum dedicated to the ingredient in Tokyo that we really became aware of how other cultures treat it. Long before provenance of food became fashionable in Britain, it was the Japanese who paid respect to its origin and treated salt with the admiration we ourselves felt. The importance of mineral balance and careful attention to structure there was obvious.

In 1997, we came back from Japan ready to perfect our own process. We named our company Halen Môn and went back to the ways that salt was made on Anglesey up until 1775 — with the help of some modern technology. Today we supply a number of the world's top 50 restaurants and chefs — from Heston Blumenthal in the UK to Dan Barber in New York.

In times gone by, salt was prized, valued and celebrated. Today, it seems to be in the news for all the wrong reasons. In the following pages, we hope to persuade you that there is much magic to be discovered in understanding this ingredient properly.

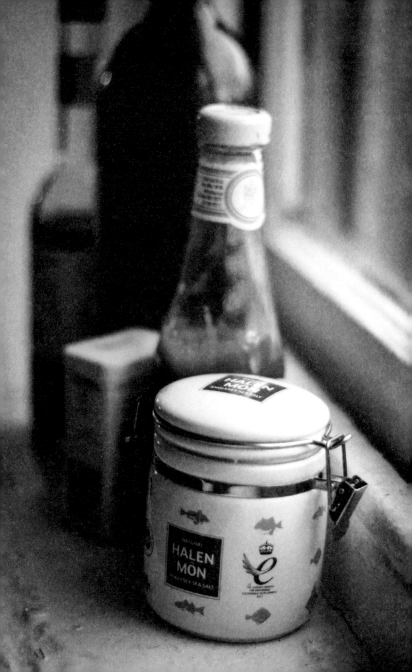

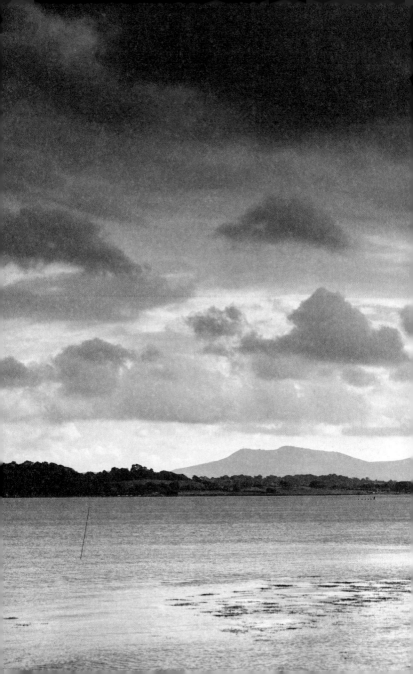

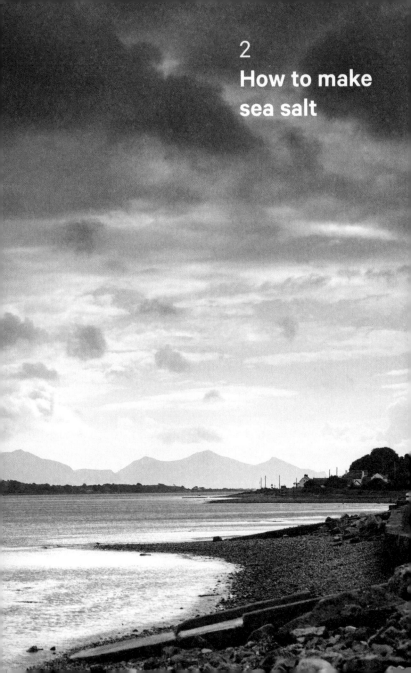

2
How to make sea salt

> A kiss without a beard
> is like an egg without salt
>
> —
>
> Dutch proverb

**All you fundamentally need to make sea salt on a small
scale is a couple of litres of clean seawater, a filter, some
heat and a saucepan. It's best to use clean seawater.
You can usually tell if seawater is clean by looking for
evidence of life — whether that be seaweed or fish — in
the body of water where you gather it.**

About 1.5 litres / 2½ pints of seawater yields around
30g / 1oz of sea salt for us, but amounts will vary a little.
Bear in mind that it feels like a lot of liquid for the amount
of salt you're left with!

(If you don't live near the sea then of course you can
still experience this magic. Dissolve some sea salt into tap
water and follow the instructions from step 5.)

You will need

— **a very clean 1.5 – 2 litre / 2½ – 3½ pint container**
an old-fashioned glass demijohn (often used for
wine-making) would be ideal and preferable to plastic,
though you can use a plastic water bottle if needed

— **a wide stainless-steel saucepan** (not an aluminium one)

— **a clean tea towel**

— **a fine sieve**

— **a shallow flat-bottomed ovenproof dish**

— **kitchen paper**

— **1.5 hours for the quick method,** 10 – 15 hours+ for the
slower method!

Instructions

1. Make sure your container is clean and doesn't smell
   tainted in any way.

2. Find the cleanest source of seawater you can and fill
   your container.

3. When you get it back to your kitchen let the seawater
   settle for a few hours. Any sand should sink to the
   bottom and even most seaweed will sink.

4. Take the sieve and put one layer of the tea towel inside
   it. Slowly pour almost all the seawater through the
   sieve and tea towel into the saucepan, leaving the last
   1cm / ½ inch in your container. Make sure that you are
   watching carefully and that you stop before the last bit

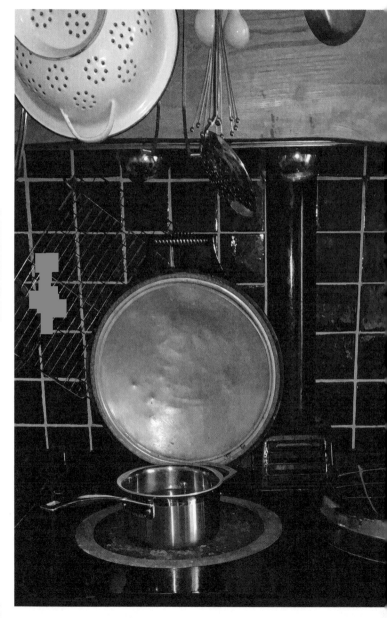

of sediment is reached. (Think of fine wine where you leave the last bit of sediment in the bottle.)

5. Put the saucepan on to a medium heat with the quick method and a low simmer with the slow method. Don't use a lid — the object is to evaporate as much as possible.

If you want quick(er) results:

6. Turn the heat up high and turn on an extraction fan in the kitchen. Open the window too if you need to; you're going to have a lot of steam!

7. Boil away at least half the starting volume, and then turn the heat down to a simmer. Do not shake or stir the pan. Then turn the heat down to the point where the pan just stops boiling — ideally very few bubbles will be visible but the source of heat will be still on.

8. When the water level reaches about one third of the original volume the heat needs to be reduced to a gentler simmer. Resist the temptation to shake or stir and watch instead.

9. This is when the magic starts to happen (we still find it magical after 22 years' practice with bigger pans!) The seawater is now strong brine and at some point you will see white specks of chalk appearing on the surface. Keep watching. Don't let the pan boil dry!

10. Some flecks will then start forming — your first crystals of sea salt. Take a few out with a spoon and have a taste (make sure you let the spoon cool first!)

11. Then leave the salt solution quietly evaporating on the lowest heat setting available. Notice that the flecks of

salt get bigger and they may sink to the bottom. When there is very little water left (enough to cover the bottom of the pan by a few millimetres) the crystals of sea salt will have formed. Turn the heat off.

12. Harvest your salt by pouring away the remaining liquid or lifting the crystals out of the liquid with a spoon and put them onto the kitchen paper. Sometimes there is a fine deposit on the side and bottom of the saucepan. This is the chalk that seashells are made from — you only want the crystals of sea salt (although both are edible).

13. Leave the crystals to dry in a thin layer on your kitchen paper for a few minutes.

14. Carefully transfer the salt crystals to the shallow dish, spread them out in a thin layer and put the dish in an oven set at a very low temperature — ideally 55−70°C / 130−160°F / GAS ½.

15. Fifteen minutes later the salt will be dry and ready to use. Keep it dry in a jar and it will last near enough forever. (Salt found in ancient Egyptian tombs is still edible today.)

For the slower method

Leave the pan at the lowest heat you can and allow the seawater to gently evaporate for many hours (10−15+), then follow the instructions from step 12.

Now to get technical

Your salt could end up as hard, soft, chalky, flaky, sludgy, or if you're lucky, shaped liked hollow upside-down pyramids. Whatever you make will be edible if the source seawater was clean.

The shape of the crystals is called 'mouthfeel' in the food industry, and is key when it comes to thinking about how we enjoy our food. Think about the coating of fine table salt on French fries tasting very different to a few perfect flakes on well-cooked roast potatoes.

From our experience, the 10 factors that can affect taste, texture and structure of your sea salt are below:

1. **Seawater source.**
   Consider how oysters taste different depending on where they're from. This is largely because of the seawater; it is the same with salt.

2. **Humidity of the air over the pan.**
   An extraction fan will make a difference. The more humidity you remove the quicker the salt forms.

3. **Speed of heating.**
   Whether you left it to blip away or have ramped up the heat. The hotter the heat, the smaller the crystals.

4. **Temperature in the pan at the top and bottom and across the surface.**
   You could try carefully baking the seawater at a low temperature for an even evaporation.

5. **The shape of your pan.**
   A tall narrow pan will work slower than a wide one due to having less surface area for evaporation.

6. **The level of liquid in the pan.**
   The liquid level goes down as the water evaporates as steam but this means the temperature goes up unless you keep reducing the source of temperature!

7. **Whether the heat source is above or below the liquid.**
   Salt crystals form slightly differently in a cooling liquid.

8. **The atmospheric pressure on the day.**

9. **The air movement over the pan.**
   A fan will speed evaporation if blown gently over the water surface but the crystal shape will change and probably be smaller.

10. **The speed at which the liquid cools**.
    Bigger crystals form on a very slowly cooling liquid so you can experiment getting the biggest crystals you can. The aim is to minimise the movement of water in the pan. Even at a low heat the hotter water at the bottom of the pan will be rising to the surface. The lower the heat the bigger the crystals — so you can control the crystal size. (We sometimes make 'diamonds of the sea' — exceptionally beautiful crystals up to 6cm wide. We still aren't 100 per cent sure why they form some days and not others — we're just very glad when they do!)

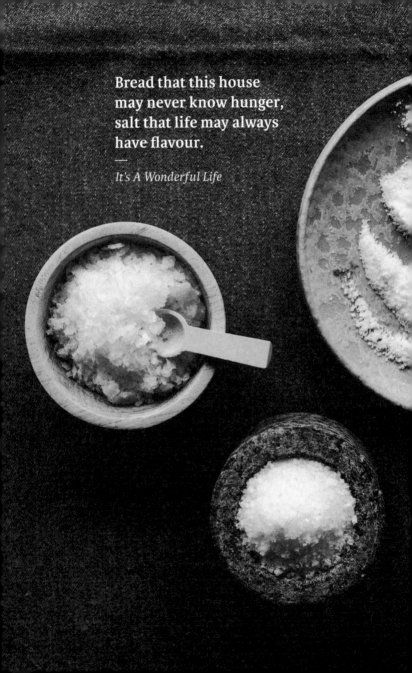

Bread that this house
may never know hunger,
salt that life may always
have flavour.

—

It's A Wonderful Life

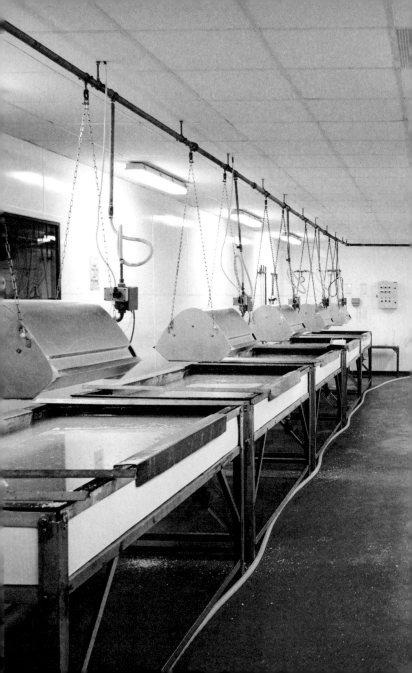

How we make sea salt on a large scale

At Halen Môn, we make about a hundred tons of sea salt a year. Most days we pump enough seawater to fill an Olympic-sized swimming pool into our holding tanks (about 20,000 litres / 35,000 pints). Atlantic seawater is about 3 per cent salt.

The water in the Menai Strait, our local water source, is very clean. Natural filtering by a mussel bed means it is even cleaner. Even so (like you using the tea towel earlier) we filter our fresh seawater to remove seaweed and sand particles larger than one micron (if you aren't familiar with microns, 10 microns is smaller than the full stop at the end of this sentence).

We pump the seawater into our evaporator, where we start to warm it up. Because we heat the seawater under a vacuum, it boils at 80°C/175°F. The freshwater steam that comes off the boiling seawater means that what's left is even saltier. Once our seawater is concentrated enough, we pump it out of the evaporator into a blending tank.

We blend the concentrated brine from different batches to the exact level of salinity we require for the next day's salt-making. Here we also add any flakes of our own sea salt that have been too small to make the grade. Then we pump the super concentrated brine into crystallisers — shallow tanks where the crystals will form.

The sea salt crystals grow on the surface of the water, until they are too heavy to float and fall into the bottom of the crystalliser. Our salt harvesters then gently scoop the crystals out of the tanks and rinse them until the right taste, texture and degree of sparkle is achieved. We then move the snowy piles of salt into low-temperature ovens to dry — but not completely. A touch of moisture keeps our crystals beautifully crisp.

We unload the dryers and pour the sea salt into large storage tubs, before packing it into our distinctive white and blue tubes and pouches. This is the salt that reaches you — anywhere, from Anglesey to Australia.

People often say to us, 'sea salt is just salt and it all tastes the same'. Clearly, we disagree. We have spent the last 20 years developing a process that makes our sea salt taste balanced and pure. Our process is, in fact, so unique that Halen Môn has become a protected food name — just like Parma ham and champagne, it can only be made in a certain place and in a certain way.

No one is surprised by wine tasting completely different depending on where the grapes come from, yet essentially they are all made from fermented grape juice. The wine world talks about terroir being crucial to the essence of the wine and the result of provenance, method of production and micro-climate. Sea salts made from different seawaters using different methods of production gives what we would term different 'merroir'.

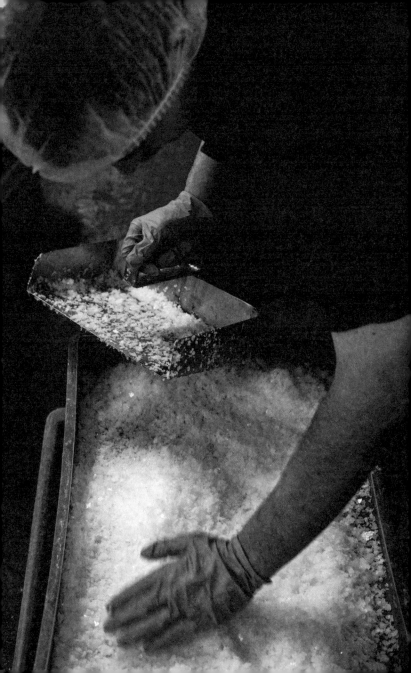

Alternative production methods
for large-scale salt-making

One of the most natural ways to make salt is by evaporating seawater in the open air (clearly in warmer climes, with less rain than in Wales!) Seawater concentrates in a shallow pond and is often moved nearer the shore into ever shallower ponds until crystals form. These are made up of both salt and all the other elements that happen to be present, so the salt may vary in colour according to where it's made. Grey salt, famous in Guérande for example, gets its hue from the clay soils that form the base of the ponds.

Another method is to boil seawater under artificial heat until almost no liquid remains. Some companies add a cheaper salt to the water to 'strengthen' the brine and cut costs. As a practice, this has been recorded in the UK since at least 1775. The final salt product can be harvested by lifting it out or draining the pan and then shovelling it out.

In the UK, most commercial salt is made using a series of vacuum evaporators to remove the water from the brine. It's done under a vacuum so the boiling point is lower and the process is more energy efficient. Usually chemicals are used to industrially strip all the other elements so that the salt becomes 99 per cent pure sodium chloride and 1 per cent moisture. This method uses massive driers to blow the salt dry and then blow it again into its packaging. When you analyse the crystals with a magnifying glass, you see that the usually naturally square salt crystals have had their corners rounded off by the drying process.

Why are sea salt crystals square?

You may have noticed that larger sea salt crystals naturally form in squares or, to be more accurate, in upside-down pyramids or layers of square crystals. At its simplest, the explanation is that the sodium chloride crystal forms around a tiny seed and grows equally at right angles as the sodium and chloride ions are equally balanced.

As each seed gets heavier with miniature salt crystals it sinks into the liquid as it overcomes surface tension. It sinks half a millimetre or so and the same process starts along each of the four surface edges. The edges act as the nucleus for crystal formation and more small squares form along each of these edges. These then sink another half millimetre and the process repeats. The crystals grow in inverted pyramids, sometimes called 'hopper crystals'.

In places such as South America, one of the most common processes is to mine ready-formed sea salt from evaporated ancient seas. Here the salt is already present and is simply gathered and sometimes only sieved before being packed.

You may have heard of *fleur de sel* (literally 'flower of salt'); for some it is regarded as the best salt money can buy. Traditionally made outdoors in parts of France, the process of concentration happens in large shallow pans placed outside. On calm, still days — the ideal conditions for salt production — the salt crystals start to form on the surface as tiny specks bonding to minute particles of chalk. These flakes are then harvested with a net and dried. To do this properly is hugely labour intensive. Reputedly the *fleur de sel* has a very delicate flavour because it contains little to no magnesium. It is this element that gives other salts a more bitter flavour as it forms at a more concentrated stage of evaporation. Unfortunately, lots of manufacturers will claim to sell *fleur de sel* but our own analysis shows it is hugely variable and only occasionally genuine.

Lastly, we wanted to mention Himalayan rock salt, though technically it hasn't come immediately from the sea. It comes from the Khewra salt mine in Pakistan, interestingly not sourced from the pristine Himalayan mountains as the name would imply, and involves conventional mining methods. Part of the attraction of this salt is its age — it is some 800 million years old — but by its nature this means when it's gone, it's gone.

It's easy enough to do a comparative tasting between types of sea salt, either tasting salts on their own or alongside something simple like cherry tomatoes. At our 'salt cote' (the traditional name for a salt-making building by the sea) we run salt tastings every day of the week, and people are always amazed at the sheer variety of flavours.

Like all flavours, salt preference is subjective. You're likely to detect a huge range of flavours in salts from different places, from bitter and acrid, sulphuric to clean, sweet to delicate. Everyone has their own preference, and different crystals sizes are suited to different foods: think of the chunky granules of rock salt on a warm pretzel, versus the fine sandy coating on a portion of fries. And we say the proof is in the eating.

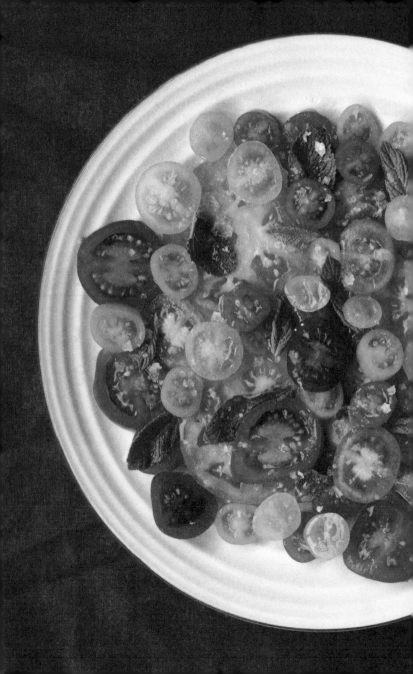

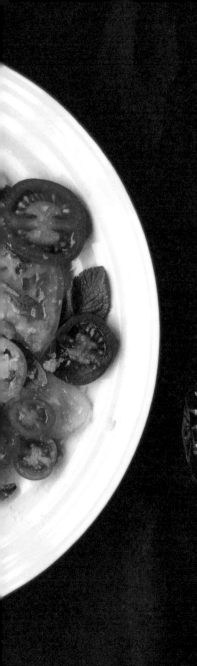
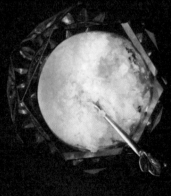

3
The essential guide to seasoning

Food needs salt. It brings dishes to life by
enhancing their flavour. It cuts through richness.
It balances sweetness. As one of the five basic
tastes, it is essential for balance. It is the most
important ingredient in the kitchen. Never trust
a cook who says they don't use salt in their food.

—

Micah Carr-Hill, former Head of Taste
at Green & Black's chocolate

**In the 1950s, despite the invention of labour-saving
devices like electric food mixers and toasters, the
average woman still spent two hours a day preparing
and cooking food (and another two hours clearing up
afterwards). Nowadays we spend around 45 minutes in
total. That's for preparation, cooking and clearing up.**

Today we buy much of our food ready-prepared. Our busy
lives, relentless schedules and the huge variety of options
for takeaways mean we don't cook from scratch nearly as
much. However, as most of us are becoming aware, this is
having consequences for our health. On average, 75 per cent
of our salt consumption is in ready-prepared foods, and,
as we peel back the plastic lid of our microwave meal,
many of us have no idea what ingredients we're putting
into our bodies. Now, with consumers pushing back and
guidelines being introduced to reduce excessive and
unnecessary amounts of salt in certain products, who
knows what other ingredients have been added to try and
enhance the flavour instead?

Previous generations, and most of our grandmothers,
seemed to know the ingredients that made up our dinners.
Somewhere along the way we have lost skills — from basic

meat preparation to bread making to the crucial understanding of how to season our food properly. Our reliance on over-processed prepared foods has made us less able to season our food confidently and competently, and when we *do* cook, many of us are wary of using any salt at all.

We're not suggesting that everyone go back to plucking their own chickens and curing their own meats (though we'd be delighted if more of us did!) but how to season food is a forgotten, essential skill that we need to be reminded of.

Our answer is simple. Make a habit of cooking from scratch and know what you're putting into your meals. Use good sea salt — you'll find it stronger so won't need quite so much — and by the time you've read this chapter, should know how to use it well.

Balancing flavour

Whether a Sunday roast or an elaborate display of a chef's 'vision and talents', we have all experienced the disappointment that comes from dining on a plate of bland food that hasn't been properly seasoned. What should be a celebratory dance on our palate often ends as nothing more than a poorly performed two-step; the food missing the peaks and valleys of flavour present in a carefully seasoned plate (an over-salted meal is equally, if not more, depressing).

Seasoning with salt should not be a random act, rather one of calculated purpose, supported by the cook's own instinct and tastes. One of the most important things to consider is adding salt at every stage of the cooking process — adding a small amount earlier on in a recipe will change the flavour in a way that adding a liberal sprinkle at the table cannot.

Layered and considerate, proper seasoning showcases not only the quality of the ingredients in the dish, but in many ways, the skill of the cook. But before we get too technical, let's take a look at our innate ability to taste.

The five tastes

— **Sweet**
— **Salty**
— **Sour**
— **Bitter**
— **Umami**

How you taste salt and flavour in your mouth

Until recently, a map of the human tongue, divided into sections of sweet, salty, sour and bitter, was widely believed to show how we interpreted food. The map, developed by Edwin Boring, has since been largely discredited. Not only can we taste all flavours all over the tongue (and taste buds are found elsewhere — in the roof of the mouth and even in the throat), Boring missed out one crucial element of our palate's profile: umami. Separate from 'salty', this is the savoury, protein-like flavour we get from things like sun-dried tomatoes and Parmesan.

It's balancing all these elements — sweet, salty, sour, bitter and umami — that makes a plate of food delicious and tells our brain that we're satisfied.

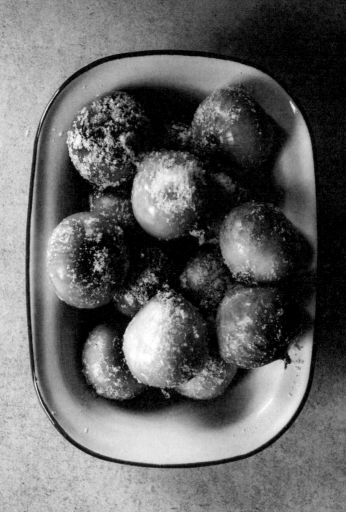

Why we use salt for cooking

— **Enhancing flavour (the primary use)**
— **Removing bitterness**
— **Drawing out water**
— **Finish and texture**
— **Preserving foods**

Salt makes foods sing by enlivening and enhancing individual flavours. Used in chocolate cookies, for example, it makes the cocoa taste more intense and chocolatey and the butter more buttery. It balances out the high-pitched sweetness of caster sugar. It suppresses bitterness (which we are hard-wired to avoid too much of); simply, it brings out savoury and sweet flavours in foods.

How salt affects food

Osmosis

Good food is the balance of flavours, and the way that salt itself works is all about balance too. The dispersal of salt through food can be explained by osmosis.

Think of vegetables sprinkled with salt that are waiting to be barbecued. Left for any longer than 10 minutes and water will appear on the surface. Salt triggers osmosis by attracting the water inside a vegetable and causing it to move toward it, through the membrane. The process of osmosis has meant that salt has entered the vegetable, and water has come out. Salt replaces some of the water content in the vegetable: softening, seasoning, flavouring and improving.

Some chefs believe in seasoning, particularly meat, in advance of cooking, to allow the *diffusion* of the salt to work its magic. When salting a chicken for example, the salt moves from the saltier environment on the skin to the less salty one inside the meat. The salt allows the heat to flow more evenly through the disrupted area. Only salt for 24 hours in advance though, otherwise you may start 'curing' the meat — essentially removing too much water — which can toughen it (think of biltong!)

Brining

The submerging of (usually) a piece of meat or poultry in a vat of salted, spiced water, brining is the ultimate way to add seasoning, as well as flavour and succulence, before cooking. The salt and water within the meat cells balance with the salt and water in the surrounding saltwater, which results in a higher concentration of salt and water in the meat, making it moist and delicious. We have a recipe for brine in the next chapter.

Preserving

When food spoils, it's not because it's old, but because bacteria and microorganisms feed on it. As we know, when used in larger amounts, salt removes water and kills bacteria, preserving food for longer and often transforming its texture and flavour. So, foods can be packed in salt and left alone for the magic to unfold. Preserved lemons are a great example of this: The lemons are cut into slices and packed tightly in jars of salt and just left to stand for three months.

Use about 250g / 1 cup flaky sea salt for around 12 lemons. Wash and slice them and place them in sterilised jars, packing the salt around them tightly. After about 90 days, the lemons can be used, rind and all, as a zesty, salty kick in many dishes from herbed couscous to winter salads.

Simple dry cures, often a mixture of salt, sugar and a few aromatics, can really transform meat and fish while preserving them at the same time. Fillets of oily fish can be transformed into an easy gravadlax in a couple of days; a side of bacon can be cured within a week, whereas a leg of prosciutto ham will generally have a whole month of curing before being hung to mature for at least 12 months.

Salt and sweet

Salt is a vital ingredient for unlocking the flavour in our food and there is no reason why this should stop at savoury. The amount we use is on a scale of course, and perhaps even more so with sweet things — when we add a scattering of salt to a home-made granola we are generally wanting to enhance the nuttiness of the cereal, whereas when we add it to popcorn or caramel we want to take it further and to taste the salt along with the sweet notes.

When something is both sweet and salty at the same time, it satisfies two cravings at once — the sugar tells us it's an energy source, and the salt is something we need to survive. Though on first thought it sounds fairly unusual, you'll find you're probably already enjoying it. Think of any sort of pickle, ketchup or chutney, the all-American favourite of peanut butter and jelly or a salted caramel chocolate.

Sugar and salt also make a good marriage for curing, as any Scandinavian will tell you. The sugar softens the cure, alleviating the harsh effects of the salt, which is why it's known as a 'soft' or 'loose' cure.

Bitterness

Salt draws out bitterness from vegetables such as aubergines before you cook them (you will also have less moisture to contend with). It also has an almost magical effect on anything naturally bitter, such as tonic water. Try it for yourself: take two glasses of tonic water. Sip one and then add a little salt. Sip it again; if you can still taste bitterness, add a little more salt. Keep sipping and adding until the tonic water tastes sweet. Then compare it to the first glass otherwise your taste buds won't believe it. Some people add a tiny pinch of salt to their coffee for this exact reason, and it has the added benefit of enhancing the flavour too.

Salt and pepper

In the West, it's very much the norm to add both salt and pepper to our food, but this certainly isn't the case around the world. Adding salt does add its own subtle flavour, but mostly it enhances what's already there. Think of a ripe, glistening tomato salad — a scattering of the good stuff makes it taste so much more of tomato. Adding pepper though, introduces an aromatic, spicy flavour all of its own. In Middle Eastern cuisines, it's often za'atar, a spice blend based around wild thyme, which is added at the table. Clearly very different to the taste of cracked black pepper.

Somewhere along the line it became usual for us to add both salt and pepper to every meal, but we'd recommend taking a moment to check whether it really is the heat of pepper you're after before reaching for the grinder.

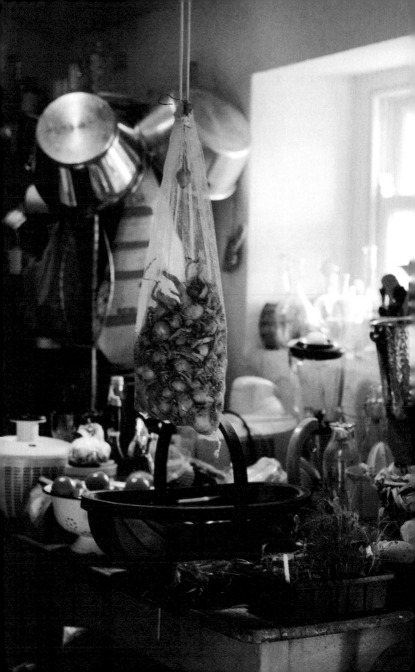

Salt to have in your kitchen

While table salt is the most common variety of cooking salt found in much of the world, we believe it doesn't belong anywhere near the kitchen. Though cheap and easy to pour from a spout, it is often laden with anticaking agents that can impart their own sour or bitter flavour to food — we discuss this in more depth in chapter 5.

As the single most important ingredient in your kitchen, we'd suggest that it's worth splashing out on sea salt rather than an acrid table version. There are many makers of quality sea salt and every coastal country has their own version.

We always have at least one finer flake and one with larger, crunchy crystals on hand. (We refer to them in our recipes as fine and flaky sea salt.) The former dissolves quickly in liquid and offers a more even distribution of flavour, while the flaky variety offers 'pops' of saltiness, which are perfect for finishing dishes.

Keep them in containers near the cooker that are easy to get to. Ideally, salt boxes or jars should be wide enough to get your hand into, and should have a lid or seal, as salt always seeks to absorb moisture. We favour a salt 'pig' (a traditional conical-shaped ceramic holder) or box — something designed to keep moisture out, rather than a salt cellar, which looks pretty for special suppers but isn't as practical.

How much salt to add

If you're following a recipe, particularly a baking recipe, take care to note the type of salt it calls for. Salts vary hugely in their shape, taste, colour and texture. Though you mightn't think it will make a difference, it may well do when it comes to *quantity*. One teaspoon of table salt will not be the same as one teaspoon of a flaked sea salt, which will be slightly stronger. You'll find some complicated tables converting different types online, but our best piece of advice would be to use the same salt(s) in your kitchen consistently. Get to know them and how much you need. If you don't have the specific type that a recipe calls for, add what you do have in small amounts, and rely on your taste buds to guide you.

In her brilliant book, *Salt, Fat, Acid, Heat*, Samin Nosrat encourages you to practise distributing salt evenly, understanding how it feels between your fingers. Baking recipes tend to be precise, but with cooking, it's as much experience as anything else that will lead you to know how much you need for a particular-sized pan of vegetables, or how many flakes to flick on to a caramel before twisting it into greaseproof paper.

Remember two more things when it comes to quantity of salt. Firstly, when boiling salted water, remember that the vast majority of the salt you add will be poured down the drain. So don't be alarmed when you are required to be liberal with your sea salt in your vat of pasta. And secondly, will there be ready-salted ingredients in your dish? Olives, anchovies, cured meats or capers all mean you will need to dial back the salt.

Good cooks taste. A lot. How much salt is needed in a dish is often determined by when it is added. It's important to try your dish at every stage. Just putting a little dab of the food on the end of a teaspoon and rolling it across your palate can help determine how much salt to add. Seasoning in different stages helps to produce food that is more refined and, ultimately, more enjoyable.

Salt is useful in almost all the stages of the cooking process. Generally speaking, it's better to add finer salt during cooking, as it delivers an even coating and dissolves quickly. Use it in anything and everything, from boiling vegetables to soups, stews, pasta, roasting vegetables and meats.

The flaky salt, however, is magnificent to add to foods when they're ready to serve as good crystals will retain their structure. Think of the crunch of flaked salt on a glistening chip, a pinch sprinkled on a cucumber salad, or a delicate quail's egg dipped in crisp smoked salt flakes. We can't think of anything better than a flake which dissolves on the tongue, flooding your mouth with a bright saline flavour. This is when flavoured salts are generally best added too.

There are, of course, exceptions to the rule of when to use different crystal sizes. One of our favourite ways to cook steak is to liberally sprinkle a good pinch of our own flaky sea salt into a very hot griddle pan. This way of cooking steak requires no fat but gives a glorious crust to the meat and prevents it from sticking.

A common mistake of the home cook is only to season at one step during the cooking process. But for a plate of food to sing, salt must be added in small doses throughout each stage of a recipe.

THE ESSENTIAL GUIDE TO SEASONING

Though it's also worth noting that when it comes to sea salt, less is more. As salt producers, we believe that while salt should be used consistently throughout most cooking processes, we should avoid the temptation to over-season. The characteristics of a good salt — its slight sweetness, minerality, clean brininess — shine through best when used in thoughtful amounts. Bland food without salt is a sad loss, but it is nonetheless still edible. But a dish that took hours to prepare will be for nothing if it's too salty.

Broadly, we recommend a three-stage approach to seasoning:

1. **The beginning**

   Think about an onion: an ingredient often characterised by layers of harsh odours and sharp tastes. If left to its own devices, cut thin and stewed without the early addition of salt, it will keep these flavours. But if just a few flakes of good salt are added, just as the onion begins to warm, something truly magical happens.

   The salt, almost instantly, expels the moisture and the sulphuric bitterness. Soon the onion's hidden identity comes alive. If allowed to gently cook, it will transform almost entirely, becoming as sweet as a perfectly ripened tomato and an ideal component for a sweet and savoury tart, a deep frittata, a rich hummus, or the foundations of a soul-satisfying bowl of onion soup.

2. **The middle**

   When most people think of layers of flavour in food they often think of the variety of ingredients used, but this is often not the true origins of nuanced flavour. Seasoning with salt in stages is the key that unlocks each ingredient's true potential.

Take for instance our tomato and onion tart. Should we fail to add the appropriate amount of salt to the pastry, or miss the opportunity to highlight the tomatoes' sweetness with a light sprinkling of salt before roasting them in the oven, our tart will inevitably be one dimensional.

Same with our onion soup: while the well-seasoned onions make a flavourful base, it would be a shame not to add any additional salt after topping the onions with a rich stock and tasting carefully. Salting in stages is essential for developing the depth of flavour that makes our food enjoyable.

3. **The end**

All good things must end, but thankfully in this case it means it's time to eat. Often, finishing a dish with a light sprinkling of flaky sea salt is key. It will help to cut through the sharpness of the tomatoes in your caramelised onion and tomato tart, and add an additional savoury crunch to the croutons that top your onion soup. It's perhaps worth noting that this instruction isn't a one-size-fits-all — especially if your meal uses a salty base, or is finished with another seasoned ingredient. A bowl of pasta with anchovies for instance, or a soy-rich stir fry, would not benefit from this final flourish. Pause before reaching for the salt.

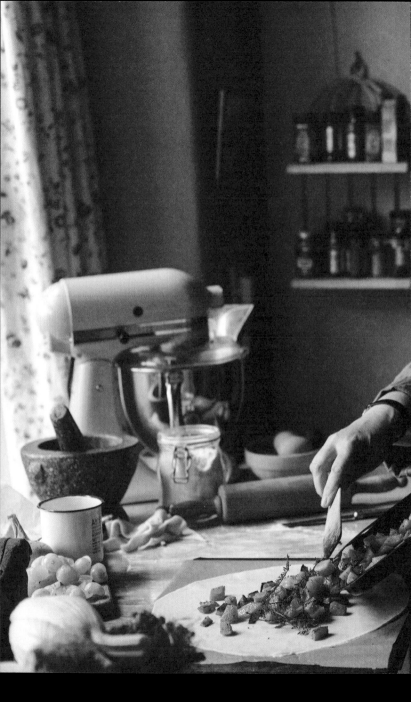

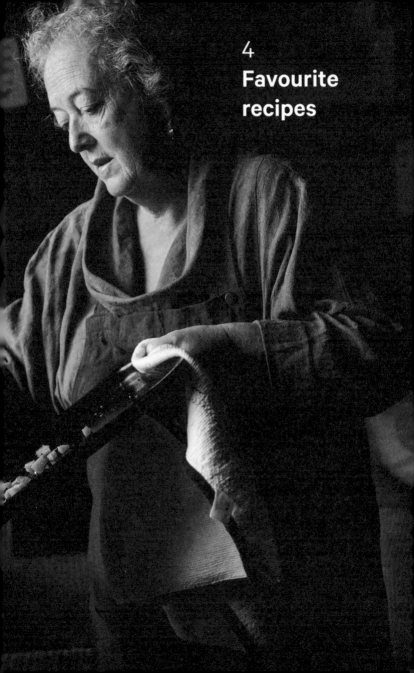

Recipes

Cooking with brine

Europeans have been cooking with brine (essentially salty water) for centuries. There are two forms it can take: the lesser-used, purified water from the ocean itself, or a home-made version, which is simply salt dissolved in water. (As a side note, we wouldn't suggest using seawater straight from the sea — it would be better (and safer) to buy a product from a reliable source that has been through some micro-filtration.)

Nowadays the general consensus is that using fresh seawater for cooking is too salty. That said, we love hearing the anecdotes told by Italian friends of local fishermen cooking up some of their fresh catch on board simply using the seawater around them. And there are chefs who swear by cooking lobsters in some of the local seawater.

Some people believe that cooking with seawater preserves even more of the trace elements than cooking with sea salt. A favourite Italian restaurant of ours in South London makes every dish with diluted purified seawater, from octopus salad to toasted seawater bread, and it's delicious. In Spain, it's not uncommon for anyone, from home cooks to Ferran Adrià, to buy purified, diluted saltwater in large bottles. The main brand, 'la sal perfecta', translates as — you guessed it, 'the perfect salt'.

A recipe for brining poultry

Aside from cooking ingredients in saltwater, 'brining' poultry in particular is a well-known technique for making it tender and moist. By submerging a chicken or turkey in salted water before cooking, it absorbs some of the liquid and salt, making it taste juicier once cooked. The below recipe is for poultry weighing around 1.5kg / 3.3lb.

2.5 litres / 10 cups water
125g / ½ cup fine sea salt
65g / ⅓ cup sugar (any type)
1 head of garlic, cut horizontally through its middle
1–2 tsp peppercorns, lightly bashed
6 bay leaves

Bring the water to a simmer in a large pan. Add all the remaining ingredients and simmer until the salt and sugar have dissolved.

Transfer the brine to a non-reactive container, such as plastic or china, and allow it to cool for a few hours.

Next, add the poultry to the container and ensure that it is covered by the liquid. Weigh it down with a large plate so that it is fully submerged.

Keep in a cool place, ideally a fridge, for 24 hours.

Drain away the brine and rinse your bird, as it can be a little too salty if you don't. Pat dry with kitchen paper, then sear in hot oil and roast in an oven using your preferred recipe.

Brined roasted root vegetables with labneh

Using a brine softens the vegetables before they're griddled and gives them a bright, spicy flavour and a deliciously tender texture, contrasting brilliantly with the smooth, cool, strained yoghurt. We use a mix of beetroot, carrots and celeriac here, but a mixture of other root veg would work just as well.

Labneh is a strained yoghurt cheese that needs a few hours to develop, but once you've spent 5 minutes setting it up, you don't need to do anything else.

Serves 4 as a side
—

For the labneh
450g / 2 cups Greek yoghurt

For the brine
250ml / 1 cup white vinegar
1 tsp fine sea salt dissolved in 50ml / 3 tbsp water
40g / 2½ tbsp caster sugar
2 bay leaves
10 peppercorns
10 coriander seeds
2 cloves

For the vegetables
300g / 2 cups mixed beetroot, unpeeled, but cleaned! (try a mix of candy, yellow and classic purple)
300g / 2 cups mixed carrots, peeled and halved lengthways
150g / 1 cup celeriac, roughly peeled and chopped into irregular triangles
a handful of basil leaves, washed and roughly torn
extra virgin olive oil, for drizzling

Start by making the labneh. Place a sieve over a bowl (leaving a few centimetres clear between the base of the sieve and the bowl) and line the sieve with cheesecloth or a couple of layers of muslin. If you don't have either, a clean tea towel will do just as well. Pour the yoghurt into the centre of the cloth and cover. Set aside for 4–6 hours, or overnight.

When the labneh has been draining for a few hours, make the brine by putting 700ml / 3 cups water and all the brine ingredients into a large saucepan. Place over a medium heat and put the beetroot into the saucepan as well. Bring to the boil and cook the beetroot at a gentle boil for 10 minutes, then remove from the brine with a slotted spoon and run them under cold water. Rub the skins from the beetroot and set aside.

Next, add the carrots and celeriac to the pan and cook them gently for 5 minutes. Remove from the pan with a slotted spoon and pat dry with kitchen paper. They will be lightly stained with pink from the beetroot, but this will look pretty when they're cooked.

Heat a griddle pan over your hob's highest heat for at least 5 minutes. Meanwhile, cut the beetroot into wedges about the size of a couple of clementine segments. Char the vegetables in batches for 3–4 minutes on each side, without moving them before you turn them (this will help clear char marks to form and a delicious smoky flavour to develop).

Remove the labneh from the cheesecloth, spread it on to a nice platter and arrange the charred vegetables over the top. Drizzle with olive oil before serving.

This makes a lovely side or add some good bread or rice for a simple lunch.

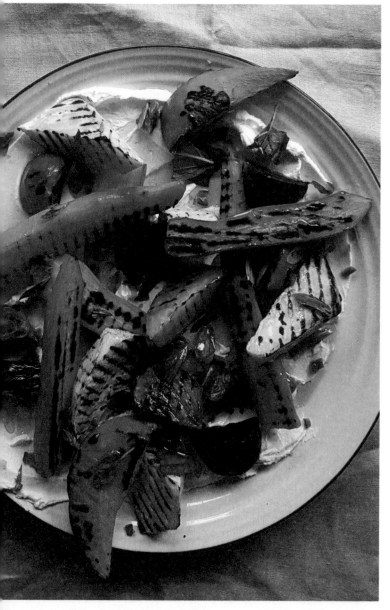

Home-made pickles

We were visiting our Japanese distributor a few years ago, a woman named Hiromi, and she kindly offered to take us to her Buddhist temple to meet the Abbot. When he heard we were salt makers, he asked his wife to bring in the special salt he used to make a particular kind of pickle that was then given to his forebears as an offering. Imagine our surprise when we saw that it was none other than Halen Môn on the offering tray!

Sea salt really comes into its own where pickles are concerned. Not only does it preserve and flavour, but it texturises too. You may be tempted to use a cheaper salt because of the quantity, but if you use sea salt it will give a much brighter flavour.

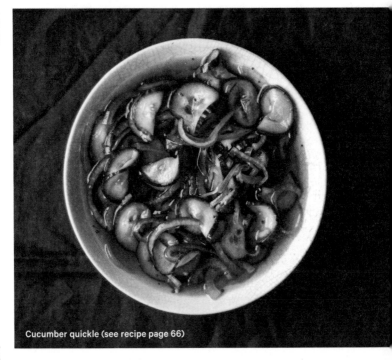

Cucumber quickle (see recipe page 66)

Pickled onions

You could also use small round shallots for this recipe.

Makes 4 × 200ml / 8fl oz jars

—

500g / 4 cups small pickling onions
50g / 3 tbsp fine sea salt
400ml / 1¾ cups malt vinegar
1 tbsp caster sugar (if you like them sweet)
1 tsp mustard seeds
a few bay leaves
a few pink or black peppercorns

Prepare your onions by putting them into a large bowl and pouring boiling water over them. Leave for 20 seconds, then tip into a colander. Return the drained onions to the bowl and tip over lots of cold water. This makes the skins easier to remove.

Make your brine by dissolving the salt in 600ml / 2½ cups warm water, then leave it to cool.

Pour the cooled brine over the peeled onions and leave overnight. If you prefer a firmer, crisper onion, then cover the onions in salt flakes rather than the brine and leave them overnight just the same. The salt will draw out moisture and make the onions even crunchier.

In the morning, drain and rinse your onions in clean water and pack into four clean, sterilised 200ml jars.

Next, add the spices and herbs to the vinegar; if you are using the caster sugar you may have to warm it slightly to dissolve. Pour the cooled spiced vinegar into the jars to cover the onions. Store at room temperature. The pickle is best left for 6 weeks to mature and will keep for up to a year.

Cucumber quickle

An even quicker pickle (quickle) is to use thinly sliced vegetables mixed with sugar and salt and covered in vinegar. We like to make cucumber and onion pickle to go with salmon or cold meats, or in a sandwich. It takes very little time to prepare and keeps for about a week in your fridge. You could also add mustard seeds and/or bay leaves along with the vinegar for more flavour.

Makes a large bowl

—

One large cucumber, thinly sliced

3 small onions, peeled and thinly sliced (if you use red ones your quickle will develop a fancy pink hue)

250g / 1¼ cups golden caster sugar

2 tbsp fine sea salt

225ml / 1 cup apple cider vinegar

Put the cut vegetables into a large bowl, sprinkle over the dry ingredients and use your hands to coat the vegetables. Pour over the vinegar and mix well. Leave in a cool place for at least 2 hours before eating. The onion will have softened and become milder.

Cherry tomato quickle

The squeaky smooth skin of tomatoes makes it difficult for the brine to penetrate the fruit and flavour them throughout, so piercing each one with a skewer helps the preserving liquid reach every curve. Serve the tomatoes alongside a cheese board or cold meats. (And just to add, the brine brings incredible flavour to a Bloody Mary.)

Makes 3 × 300ml / 12fl oz jars

—

200ml / ¾ cup apple cider vinegar
5 tsp fine sea salt
2½ tsp caster sugar
the zest of ½ lemon
500g / 2½ cups whole cherry tomatoes, each one pierced
    a couple of times with a skewer or needle
1 tsp fennel seeds
2 garlic cloves, peeled and finely sliced
1 red chilli, deseeded and finely sliced
6 tbsp extra virgin olive oil

Pour the vinegar and 200ml / ¾ cup water into a saucepan. Add the salt, sugar and lemon peel and warm over a medium heat, stirring to dissolve the sugar and salt until no crystals are visible. Remove from the heat and allow to cool for at least 30 minutes.

Toss the pierced tomatoes in a bowl with the fennel seeds, garlic and chilli. Pour over the cooled vinegar mixture and allow to stand at room temperature for 6 hours or overnight, covered with a tea towel.

Divide the pickled tomatoes and the pickling liquid between the sterilised jam jars and top each jar with 2 tablespoons of olive oil before screwing on the lid. Keep in the fridge for up to a month.

Home-made salted butter

Traditionally, dairy maids would heavily salt their butter to store it, rinsing it in fresh water when they wanted to use it. Thanks to fridges, there's no need for us to salt our butter quite so heavily now, though of course we add a little for flavour.

You can start this with kids if you like, getting them to shake the cream in a tightly sealed jar, transferring it to your food mixer when they get tired!

We always use organic cream for making butter. If you're going to the trouble of making butter, we think it's a good idea to start with the best ingredients, especially with dairy.

You can also add a flavoured salt to the raw cream for something a little different — our favourites are roasted garlic salt for chicken, fish and bread; smoked salt for baked potatoes and roasted tomatoes, and vanilla salt for maple syrup butter pancakes.

Be sure to keep the buttermilk produced by this recipe — it's delicious in the soda bread recipe on page 70.

Makes a 250g / 8oz pat of butter (and delicious buttermilk)
—

750ml / 3 cups organic double cream
1 tsp flaky sea salt (or flavoured sea salt)

Put a mixing bowl into your fridge to chill.

Use a whisk attachment on your food mixer, or an electric hand whisk to beat the cream. After around 15 minutes of beating the cream will begin to start looking like butter and the sound will change to a sort of sloshing.

Drain the cream into a clean sieve set over a bowl. The leftover liquid — buttermilk — can be used in a salad dressing or our simple soda bread recipe.

Put the butter from the sieve into a clean, cold bowl and whisk again for a minute to get rid of any excess buttermilk. Then wash the butter in ice-cold water, squeezing it between traditional wooden butter pats (or your hands!) to remove more liquid.

Finally, add the sea salt. Make a well in the centre of the butter and knead it until incorporated. Shape it however you like (you could use cutters if you're doing this with kids) and chill until firm.

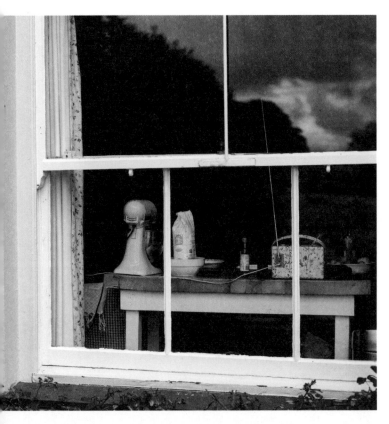

Simple soda bread

In the spirit of Do, we wanted to include a recipe to use the by-product from the butter recipe: buttermilk. This bread is a staple in our house; it comes from some good friends of ours in Dublin. Spread a warm slice with thick home-made butter (see page 68) and pickled tomatoes (page 67), or a slick of cream cheese and a slice of salmon.

Makes 1 loaf

—

250g / 2 cups wholemeal / whole-wheat flour
200g / 1⅔ cups plain flour
1 tsp bicarbonate of soda, sieved
1 tsp fine sea salt
1 egg
about 350ml / 1½ cups buttermilk
1 tsp honey
a small handful of oats

Preheat the oven to 200°C / 400°F / GAS 6. Lightly oil a 450g / 1lb loaf tin.

Mix the flours, bicarbonate of soda and salt together in a bowl.

In a separate bowl, mix the egg, buttermilk and honey, then add this to the flour. You're looking for a soft dough. You may need to add a little more buttermilk if the dough seems too stiff but it should not be too wet or sticky.

Put the dough into your prepared tin and finish with a sprinkle of oats on top.

Bake for 45–50 minutes. You'll know it's done if it sounds hollow when you tap the bottom of the loaf. For a soft crust, wrap it in a clean tea towel as soon as it comes out of the oven. Leave to cool before slicing.

FAVOURITE RECIPES

Seawater crackers

These are everything you want a cracker to be: savoury, salty and pleasingly neutral.

Makes around 24

—

200g / 1⅔ cups plain flour
1 tsp flaky sea salt, plus extra for sprinkling
1 tsp baking powder
2 tbsp extra virgin olive oil

Preheat the oven to 180°C / 350°F / GAS 4. Measure the plain flour and a teaspoon of sea salt in a mixing bowl then use a sieve to sift the baking powder into the same bowl, working out any clumps. Make a well in the centre and pour in 100ml / ½ cup cold water and the olive oil. Use a knife to 'cut' the water and oil into the flour, and continue to use the knife to mix until a shaggy ball of dough forms. Use your hands to bring the mixture together. Flatten the dough into a rough rectangle, then place it between two 30 × 30cm / 12 × 12in sheets of baking parchment. Roll the dough out to about 2mm thick with a rolling pin.

Lift away the top sheet of parchment and use it to line a large baking sheet. Use a round drinking glass or pastry cutter to cut 6cm / 2in rounds from the dough and carefully lift the rounds on to the baking sheet — the crackers won't spread as they cook so don't worry if they are closely packed together.

Prick each cracker with a fork a few times then sprinkle generously with flaky sea salt. Bake in the oven for 30 minutes, until a very pale gold. Remove the crackers from the oven to cool and crisp on a wire rack. They may seem soft but will harden. Store in an airtight container for up to a week. Eat with cheeses and pickles (see page 64).

The sweet savoury depth of a tomato tarte tatin, a glistening plate of fresh Santorini tomatoes alongside a bowl of pasta, the umami moreishness of a rich tomato sauce atop a crisp pizza, the satisfying tang of a pickled cherry tomato in a sandwich, we find that salt is especially vital when it comes to tomatoes. And none of these dishes would sing quite like they do without it. The next three recipes each contain tomatoes ... And salt.

Salt-spritzed pizza dough

When making pizza, we use a brine spray of about 10 per cent salinity, which makes for a deliciously crisp pizza crust. This technique can also be used whenever you want a good crust on bread. Spray the dough before it goes in the oven, and then again when it's in to alter the humidity.

To make your own brine spray, dissolve 2 tsp fine sea salt in 100ml / ½ cup water and pour it into a spray bottle. Keep it in the fridge. The brine is also great spritzed on salads for an even distribution of seasoning.

Makes 2 sharing pizzas or 4 individual ones
—

For the pizza dough
500g / 4 cups strong white bread flour
325ml / 1⅓ cups lukewarm water
1 tsp caster sugar
1 × 7g fast-action packet of yeast
4 tbsp olive oil, plus a little extra for the bowl
½ tsp fine sea salt

For a good tomato sauce
1 tbsp olive oil
3 garlic cloves, finely sliced
1 × 400g can chopped tomatoes
½ tsp sugar (any type)
a good pinch of fine sea salt
a pinch of black pepper
a small bunch of basil, leaves picked and stalks discarded
**   (keep a handful of leaves for the pizza topping)**

For topping (optional)
2 × 125g balls of buffalo mozzarella

Start by making the pizza dough. Sift the flour and salt on to a clean work surface and make a well in the middle. In a jug, mix the lukewarm water with the sugar, yeast and oil and set aside for a few minutes.

Pour the water into the well and use a fork to draw the flour in from the sides, gradually bringing more flour to the centre and eventually bringing the dough together in a ball with floured hands. Knead on your work surface for about 10 minutes until you have a smooth, springy dough.

Place in a lightly oiled bowl and cover with a damp tea towel. Set aside in a warm place to rise for about an hour. The dough will double in size.

While the dough is rising, make the tomato sauce by warming the olive oil in a frying pan over a medium heat. Fry the garlic until it's just starting to turn golden, then pour in the chopped tomatoes and stir in the sugar and salt. Bring to a gentle simmer, then add the black pepper and half the basil leaves and turn the heat down to low. Cook for half an hour to reduce and concentrate the flavour.

Heat the oven to 240°C / 475°F / GAS 9, or as high as it will go. Warm two large baking trays on the shelves in your oven at the same time.

Divide the pizza dough into two or four evenly sized balls, and roll each one out to about 5mm / ¼in thick. Spread a tablespoon of tomato sauce from the centre of each pizza base, leaving 1.5cm / ½in around the sides. You can add some cheese on top here if you like.

Lightly dust the warmed oven trays with flour and slide each pizza on to them. Give the pizzas a good spray of brine and then put them into the oven. Once in, spray again, but don't burn yourself. Cook the pizzas for 6–8 minutes, until golden, bubbling and with a perfect crust!

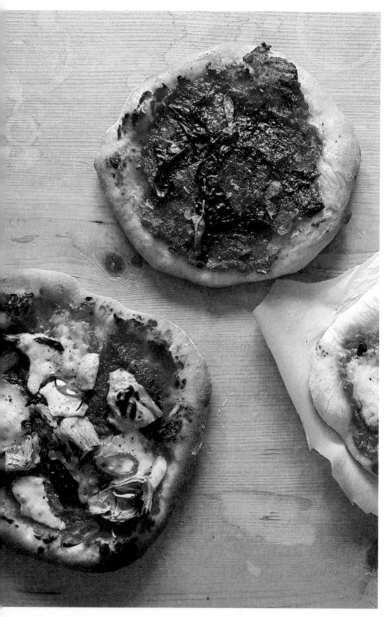

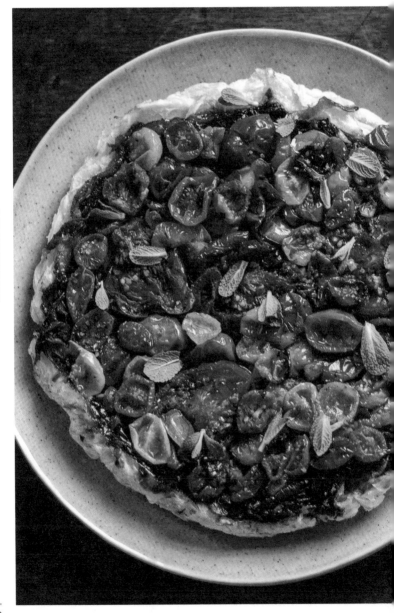

Tomato and red onion tart

In this recipe, salt is used in a few ways: sprinkled on the raw cut tomatoes it helps to dehydrate the fruit and concentrate the sugars in the oven; it draws moisture from the onions, softening them as they cook; and a final pinch of flaky sea salt adds a layer of crunch to the sweet tomatoes.

Serves 4, generously

—

1kg / 2lb 2oz tomatoes, of all shapes and sizes
¾ tsp fine sea salt
black pepper
3 tbsp extra virgin olive oil
4 red onions, finely sliced
2 garlic cloves, finely sliced
100g / ½ cup spinach, washed
grated zest of 1 lemon
1 sheet of puff pastry, 32cm × 24cm / 12½in × 9 ½in
a pinch of flaky sea salt

Preheat the oven to 120°C / 250°F / GAS ½.

Halve the tomatoes around their middles and arrange on a roasting tray. Sprinkle over half a teaspoon of sea salt and a grinding of black pepper. Place in the middle of the oven for 1½–2 hours but keep an eye on the smaller cherry tomatoes as they'll cook much more quickly. The tomatoes are done when their skins are blistered but not burnt.

While the tomatoes are cooking, heat a 23cm / 9in oven-proof frying pan over a medium heat and add a splash of olive oil.

Add the red onions and ¼ teaspoon of sea salt and cook, stirring regularly for 8–10 minutes, until the onions are soft and translucent. Add the garlic and cook for another minute or so before adding the spinach and lemon zest. Cook for a couple more minutes until the spinach wilts and becomes bright green and glossy. Take off the heat and drain any excess moisture through a sieve, pushing the spinach down with the back of a wooden spoon. Wipe the pan down with kitchen paper to dry, then rub a little olive oil around the sides. Set aside for later.

When the tomatoes have had their time, remove from the oven then turn it up to 180°C / 350°F / GAS 4. Pour a little more olive oil (about 1 tablespoon) into the bottom of the frying pan. Place the tomatoes cut-side down over the base of the pan (don't worry if there is some overlap). Arrange the onion and spinach mixture on top, then cut a sheet of pastry just larger than the rim. Lay the pastry over the spinach and tomato mix and pinch the sides in, tucking it around the spinach and tomatoes.

Place in the oven for 25–30 minutes, until the pastry is deep golden and has puffed up. Allow the tart to cool for 5 minutes before running a spatula around the edge to loosen the sides, then place a slightly larger plate over the top. Holding the pan and plate together with an oven-gloved hand on each side, bravely flip the pan over and give it a sharp knock to loosen any sticky tomatoes.

Sprinkle over a pinch of flaky salt and serve with a green salad (and a spoonful of the cherry tomato quickle if you like, see page 67).

Tomato panzanella

Panzanella is an Italian bread salad that's perfect for the height of summer when the gluts of tomatoes are almost overwhelming and it's too hot to do any real cooking. The salt draws the juices from the tomatoes, intensifying their flavour and bringing new life to stale bread. It also creates a dressing of sorts for the salad; simply finish with good olive oil.

Serves 4
—

1 shallot, finely chopped
2 tsp red wine vinegar
350g / ¾lb mixed tomatoes, larger ones sliced into wedges
    and smaller ones halved around the middle
1 tsp flaky sea salt, plus extra for sprinkling
2 large slices of stale, coarse-crumbed bread, torn into chunks
1 tsp capers, rinsed and dried
a small bunch of basil, leaves picked
3 tbsp extra virgin olive oil

Mix the shallot and vinegar together in a small bowl and set aside for 15 minutes.

Toss the tomatoes with the salt in a large mixing bowl and add the remaining ingredients. Toss again. Add the shallot vinegar and allow the flavours to mingle and the bread to soften in the tomato juices for half an hour before serving with a sprinkle of flaky salt.

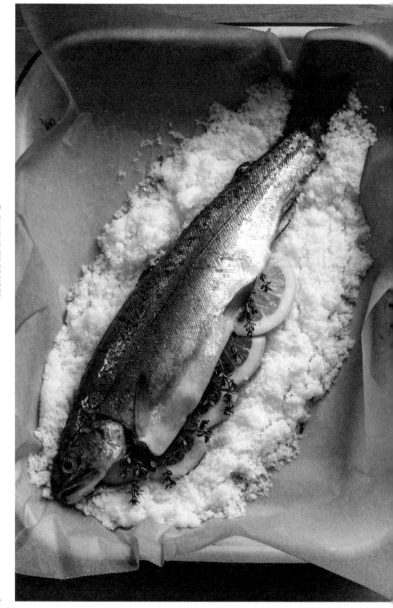

Salt-baked fish

For centuries, this method of cooking was reserved for the few who could afford such flagrant use of a precious commodity. Recipes for salt-baking have been used for thousands of years in many parts of Europe, the salt-rich coast of Africa and even as far east as China. Closer to home, many of us shy away from this method, assuming (quite logically) that baking a whole fish encased in salt would result in an overly salty supper. But actually, salt acts as a wonderful conductor of heat, dispersing dry heat evenly while retaining all of the moisture contained naturally in the flesh of the fish; all the while imparting a beautiful brininess throughout. The recipe is easy to master and a joy to eat. You can use the same technique for veg too — try beetroot or celeriac.

Many different species of fish are excellent candidates for salt-baking; we always use what's local and sustainable. For this recipe, we'd recommend a round fleshy fish, such as coley, pollack or trout. We're particularly enjoying coley at the moment because it has a lovely delicate sweetness and a flaky texture similar to that of cod.

Serves 3–4
—

1 round, fleshy fish (see above), about 30cm / 12in long, weighing roughly 1kg / 2lb (have your fishmonger gut and scale the fish, being sure to remove the fins)
1kg / 2lb fine or kosher sea salt

To serve
lemon wedges
fresh herbs
olive oil
black pepper
green salad
good crusty bread

Heat the oven to 180°C / 350°F / GAS 4.

In a medium-sized bowl mix 1kg / 2lb fine or kosher sea salt with 100ml / ½ cup water and one egg white. Once mixed it will look much like wet sand. Fill the cavity of your fish with slices of fresh lemon, and whatever herbs you fancy.

Line a baking tray with parchment. Place a handful of the salt sand on a baking tray, spreading it out in a thin, even layer, making sure to flatten it out to the full length of the fish. Place the fish on top of the sand mass and tightly pack the remaining mixture all the way around the fish ensuring there are no perforations.

Place in the oven for 25 – 30 minutes, or until crisp. Remove it and pierce the now hardened dome with a thermometer in the thickest part of the fish, nearest the head. It should reach 58°C / 136°F. If not, return it to the oven and check it again in another 5 minutes.

Once cooked, remove from the oven and allow the fish to rest for 5 minutes inside the salt crust. With a sharp knife cut all the way around the fish and gently remove the dome of salt. The skin should come off in one piece, if you pull it from tail to head. Peel the cooked fillets off the bone and dress with a squeeze of lemon juice, herbs, a glug of olive oil, and for good measure a crank of pepper.

Serve with a crisp green salad and some good bread.

Salted jacket potatoes

Few things are as comforting as a jacket potato. Often found in the American South at roadside steakhouses, their version of the jacket is lacquered with oil then liberally rolled with salt prior to baking. The salt tightens the skin making it crunchy, while the interior becomes light, fluffy, and nicely seasoned.

**1 medium-sized starchy potato, such as Maris Piper or
   King Edward, per diner
olive oil, for brushing
flaky sea salt**

Set your oven to 220°C / 425°F / GAS 7. The high heat will help create the crackling exterior.

With a fork, pierce the skin all the way around the potatoes. Brush the skin with olive oil then immediately roll the potato through a dish of flaky sea salt. Allow the potatoes to bake on a tray for about an hour depending on size. Let them cool for a minute or two, then slit them lengthwise.

Garnish with whatever you fancy. Keeping true to American tradition, we recommend a dollop of soured cream, a spoonful (or two) of fried bacon bits, and slices of spring onion.

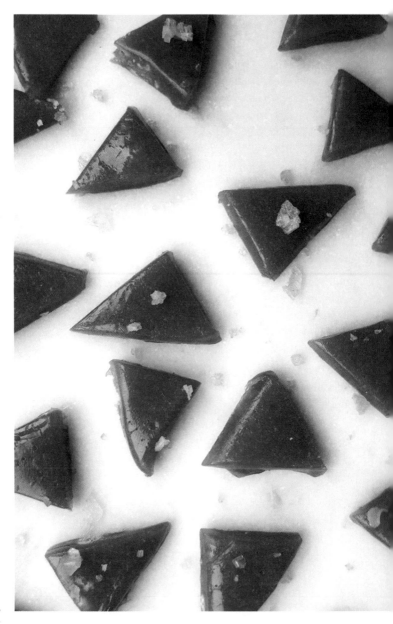

Salted caramel chews

Our friends at Fran's Caramels in Seattle make their soft, buttery caramels and then dip them in rich 39 per cent milk chocolate, finishing with our very own smoked sea salt. If you ever get the chance to try one, seize it, because there is nothing quite like them.

That said, this recipe comes fairly close to the fudgy deliciousness of Fran's. You will need greaseproof paper for wrapping the chews, a pastry brush and a sugar thermometer. If you're feeling generous, these make the most delicious gift.

Makes 36 chews

—

200g / 1 cup caster sugar
50g / ⅛ cup golden syrup
275ml / 1 cup double / heavy cream
100g unsalted butter, cut into cubes
1 tsp vanilla extract or paste
1 heaped tsp flaky sea salt
a good pinch of smoked sea salt, for sprinkling

Begin by lining a 20cm / 8in square cake tin with greaseproof paper.

Measure the caster sugar, golden syrup and 3 tablespoons of cold water into a large saucepan. Tilt the pan so there are no dry patches of sugar visible. Place the pan over a medium heat and continue to tilt (don't stir), until all of the sugar has melted. Remove the pan from the heat as soon as the sugar has melted and there are no sugar crystals visible. If you spot any on the sides of the pan, use a wet pastry brush to brush them down towards the melted sugar mixture and continue to heat gently until all of the sugar has melted.

Pour the cream into a separate saucepan and heat gently over a low heat until it just starts to steam. Using a hand whisk, whisk the butter into the cream and remove from the heat. Put on oven gloves to pour the cream and butter mixture into the sugar pan (carefully, as it will bubble up), then clip a sugar thermometer on to the side of the pan and return the pan to a medium heat. Cook until the mixture reaches 110°C / 230°F on the sugar thermometer (about 8–10 minutes), then remove from the heat and quickly stir in the vanilla and sea salt. Wearing oven gloves again, pour the caramel mixture into the prepared tin and sprinkle the top with a little smoked sea salt. Chill in the fridge overnight.

The following day, remove the tin from the fridge and lift the caramel from the tin on to a chopping board. Using a sharp knife dipped in hot water, slice the caramel into individual 2cm / 1in square chews. Wrap each chew in greaseproof paper to give as gifts or eat straightaway. Eat within a week.

Sea-salted chocolate truffles

In recent years, it's become rather fashionable to add salt to chocolate. We supply our sea salt to makers, large and small, all over the world, including Green & Black's, who kindly shared this delicious sea-salted chocolate truffle recipe with us.

Madeira is a fitting tipple to add to this recipe, as it too has a relationship with the sea. Centuries ago sailors discovered that white wine from the island of Madeira would transform into a dark, richly flavoured wine after weeks of the sun beating down upon the deck and the gentle rocking motion of the ship on the waves. This inspired a style of fortified wine that has complex flavours of raisins, walnuts, coffee and spices, which marry beautifully with the caramel notes in high-cocoa milk chocolate. The delicate flakes of pure sea salt help to accentuate these flavours and cut through the richness.

There's no need to create extra washing up by melting the chocolate over a bain-marie (as many recipes suggest), so long as you are careful never to let the pan get too hot once the chocolate has been added. Use a low heat and take your time, and you will be rewarded with a delicious recipe with minimal fuss. This recipe makes enough for around 15 truffles — 3 to try and 12 to wrap up for a present. Feel free to experiment with the recipe, trying different alcohols in place of the Madeira.

Makes 15 truffles

—

2 tbsp sweet Madeira
a large pinch of flaky sea salt
200g / 8oz good-quality milk chocolate
100g / ½ cup cocoa powder

Put the Madeira, 4 teaspoons of water and the sea salt into a small saucepan and bring to just below simmering point.

Remove from the heat. Break the chocolate into pieces and add them to the saucepan, stirring continuously until smooth. If after a minute of stirring you still have unmelted pieces of chocolate, place the saucepan back on a very low heat for 10 seconds before removing and continuing to stir. Repeat if necessary. Pour the smooth mixture into a bowl and leave in the fridge until fully set, a minimum of 6 hours.

Sift the cocoa powder into a large bowl and set aside. Remove the truffle mix from the fridge, and use a teaspoon to scoop out pieces and roll them into balls using your hands — they should be about 2.5cm / 1in wide. Roll the truffles in the cocoa powder until completely covered, and keep in the fridge until ready to serve.

To serve, remove the truffles from the fridge and shake off the excess cocoa powder, 3 or 4 truffles at a time. Place on a serving plate and allow about 20 minutes to bring them to room temperature.

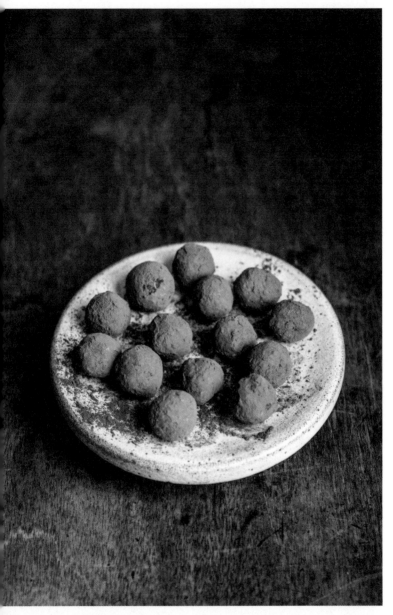

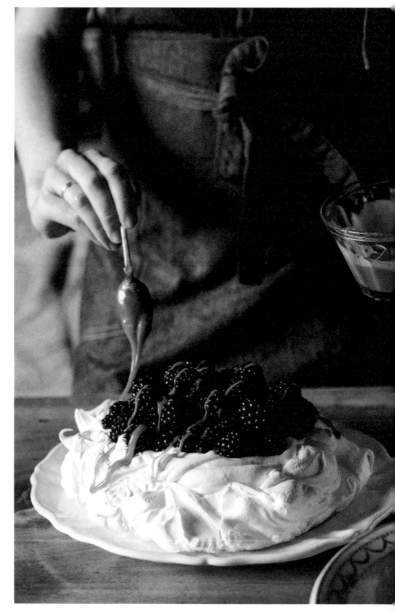

Salted caramel sauce

It's hard to believe that our very favourite combination of flavours is such a new sensation, but it's said to have been invented only 40 years ago in Brittany, when a chef used traditional French salted butter for his sweets, and accidentally stumbled across something truly brilliant. This is that golden deliciousness in liquid form.

Makes about 200ml / 1 cup

—

100g / ½ cup caster sugar
60g / ¼ cup unsalted butter, cut into cubes
50ml / ¼ cup double / heavy cream
½ tsp fine sea salt

Measure the sugar into a saucepan and pour over 3 tablespoons of water. Tilt the pan so that there are no dry patches of sugar visible. Place over a medium heat and keep an eye on the pan until all the sugar has melted. You don't want it to be boiling furiously, but a gentle simmer while the sugar melts is fine. Meanwhile, use a wet pastry brush to brush any visible sugar crystals down from the sides of the pan. This will prevent the sauce from crystallising at a later stage.

When the sugar has completely melted and turned a dark golden / light amber colour, remove from the heat and whisk in the unsalted butter to melt. Add the cream and sea salt and return the pan to the heat. Bring to the boil and continue to boil for 1 minute before pouring into a sterilised jar. Cover and keep in the fridge for up to 2 weeks.

Flavoured sea salts

When we first started our business, we thought only of making pure white sea salt, there would be none of these new-fangled flavours for us. But we soon found that people loved the idea of something quick and easy to sprinkle on food just before serving. Adding a flavoured salt to a dish adds a rather considered finish, and a pinch can look very pretty on a plate of food.

Our first seasoned-salt recipe was based on a French idea for disguising the taste of rotting meat — or for preserving it, depending on who you ask. It's a mix of nine organic spices and it works very well seasoning roasted meats and vegetables as they cook, and also as a cure, when mixed with sugar, for gravadlax.

Below are a couple of recipes, but you can easily come up with your own ideas; think of what you cook most often and what would be nice alongside.

Try adding chilli powder — perhaps more than one type so you can enjoy the waves of flavour. Cumin will add an earthy note. Grated citrus peel won't last very long but its essential oils and texture add a piquancy to a salad or roast chicken when mixed with a finer flaked sea salt and sprinkled just before eating. Spring's wild garlic is beautiful with a bright sea salt, or perhaps try aromatic whole pink peppercorns mixed with salt in a grinder for a clean flavour hit.

As a general guide, we've found that strong flavours such as chilli should be no more than 10 per cent of the overall mix, but herbs and citrus can be up to 20 per cent.

Consider how ingredients will look in a jar or grinder, as they make lovely home-made gifts too.

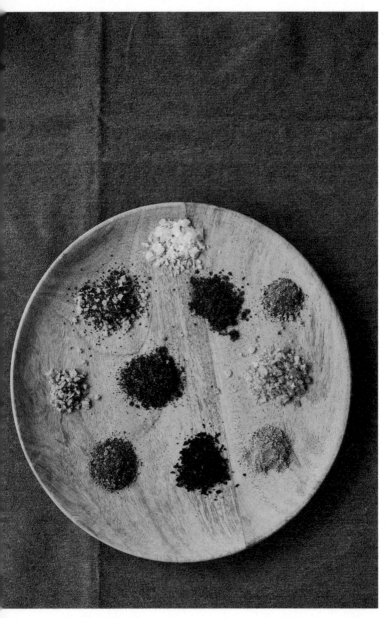

Sweet spiced salt

This spice blend will add depth and body to Mexican and Indian dishes, and is delicious sprinkled over roasted carrots or squash. Stir into curries, tagines or black beans for a rounded, sweet/savoury flavour boost.

Makes about 150g / ½ cup

—

1 tbsp cumin seeds
1½ tsp coriander seeds
½ tsp green peppercorns (or ¼ tsp black peppercorns)
¼ tsp ground cinnamon
100g / 3oz flaky sea salt

Toast the cumin, coriander and peppercorns in a dry frying pan until they appear light golden and smell fragrant. Pulse the toasted spices in a food processor a few times until they start to break down before tipping in the cinnamon and salt. Whizz again to combine before decanting into a jar and covering with a lid. Use within a year for the most intense flavour from the spices.

Rosemary salt

This is a revelation sprinkled on top of chips or roast potatoes, but is just as good to season roast chicken or robust green vegetables, such as kale or purple sprouting broccoli. Don't be tempted to try and chop the rosemary in the food processor — unless you have a very powerful model it will only bruise the leaves rather than chop them.

Makes about 120g / ½ cup

—

4 rosemary, sprigs, leaves picked and finely chopped
100g / 3oz flaky sea salt

Whizz the hand-chopped rosemary and salt together in a food processor to combine before tipping it all on to a parchment-lined baking sheet. Allow the mixture to dry at room temperature for 4 hours, or overnight, before scooping into a jar. Cover with a lid and use within a year.

Dukkah

Another favourite recipe in our house is a home-made dukkah — an Egyptian mix of nuts, spices and seeds, toasted and mixed together. The mix is delicious when devoured with good bread and oil at the beginning of a meal, sprinkled on your fried eggs in the morning, or stirred through pasta or quinoa.

There are many recipes for this blend but most include nuts of some sort, usually hazelnuts, together with sesame seeds, coriander and cumin.

Makes about 120g / 1 cup

—

2 tbsp sesame seeds
1 tbsp coriander seeds
1 tbsp cumin seeds
1 tbsp fennel seeds (optional)
100g / 3oz walnuts / hazelnuts
1 tsp fine sea salt (or more to taste)

Toast the seeds in a heavy-based frying pan for a few minutes until fragrant. Set them aside to cool and then toast the nuts in the same way, keeping a close eye so that they don't catch and burn.

Use a pestle and mortar to grind the seeds to release some of their flavour. Then add the nuts and grind until you have the texture of crushed biscuits — you want to keep some bite.

Pour the mix into a bowl, add the salt and mix well. Taste and add more if you like. The dukkah will keep in a sealed jar for up to a month.

Salt dough for crafting (not eating!)

A classic rainy-day activity, this dough is not for eating but for crafting into simple shapes which can then be baked and painted. It's a great thing to do with children. At Christmas try making beads or simple shapes to hang on a tree or branch for decoration. Use cutters, moulds and easy templates. Chances are, you'll have everything you need for this already.

> **2 cups plain flour**
> **1 cup table salt (don't waste anything nice on this!)**
> **1 cup water**

Heat your oven at 100°C / 215°F / GAS ½ and line a baking tray with greaseproof paper.

Mix the flour and salt in a large bowl. Add the water and stir until it comes together in a clean ball. Mould into your shapes of choice. If making decorations to hang remember to leave a hole for a ribbon.

Put your finished items on to the lined baking sheet and pop in the oven for 3 hours or until solid.

Leave to cool and then paint. Thread them with ribbons or cotton for hanging.

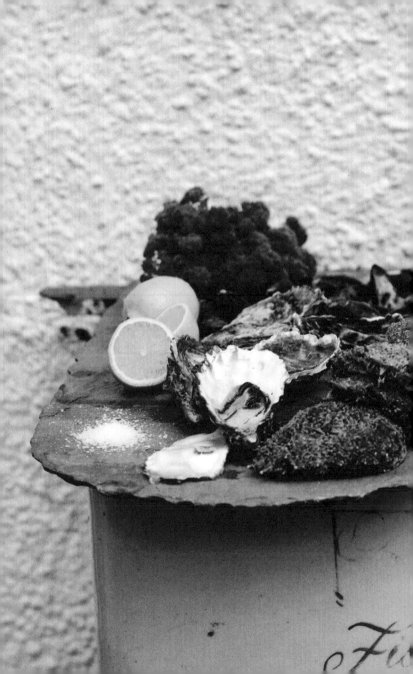

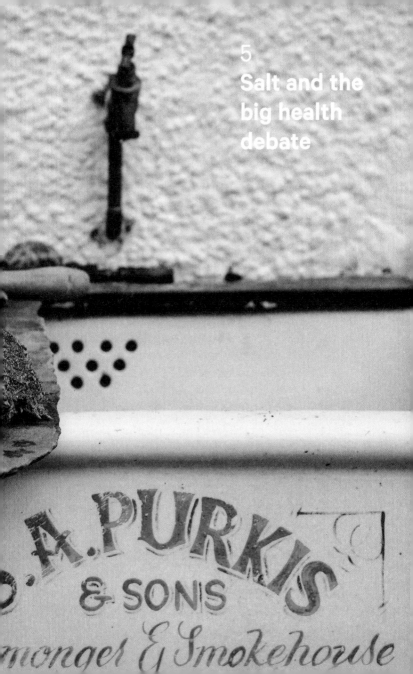

5
Salt and the
big health
debate

> Give neither counsel nor salt
> till you are asked for it
>
> —
>
> English proverb

Can salt ever be good for you?

This is the big question that a book extolling the magic of sea salt must address. And this chapter on salt and health has been the most difficult to write because, understandably, it's a rather emotive topic.

Being sea salt makers, we can be accused of bias so we have called on the help and advice of medical friends and colleagues so that we remain as objective as possible. That said, we don't purport to give health advice — only to highlight the importance of salt (and sea salt) to our survival, as well as the dangers of eating too much of it.

Our research began over 20 years ago, when we first started our business. A family business with strong ethical values, we knew we didn't want to make something that wasn't good. What we discovered is what we will begin with: a simple, two-fold starting point.

1. **The body needs salt to function**
2. **The body cannot make or store salt**

It is startling how much our bodies depend on salt for normal day-to-day functioning. It is essential for digestion, for example. It prevents dehydration. Most importantly, it is needed in cell-to-cell communication helping to keep our heart pumping and our internal organs running efficiently. And it isn't just the sodium in salt that we need for this, it's other minerals too, potassium, magnesium and calcium — all found in sea salt — that help carry out the proper functioning at cellular and molecular level.

Think of each cell (we have about 37 billion per adult) like a battery communicating with other batteries by passing an electric current between them. To get technical, each cell communicates with the aid of a different sodium and potassium balance between what is inside and outside the cell. Sodium levels are 10 times higher outside cells and potassium levels are 30 times higher inside cells. The concentration differences between potassium and sodium across cell walls create an electrochemical gradient known as the 'membrane potential'. Tight control of this requires large amounts of energy. Magnesium and calcium are also involved in the process. Together, these four elements, calcium, sodium, potassium and magnesium, are actually the most abundant minerals in the human body.

On the whole, our kidneys regulate our salt balance. You know how thirsty you can get when you eat something salty? When we drink to quench our thirst, our kidneys flush out the excess salt we have consumed. Changing our salt intake affects levels of aldosterone and glucorticoids, the hormones that rhythmically control the body's salt and water balance.

Too much of the white stuff puts more pressure on our kidneys to regulate our finely tuned systems — and excessive salt intake is one of the primary causes of high blood pressure, strokes and diabetes. But how much is too much?

In recent years, government campaigns have encouraged the UK population to reduce their salt intake and, by doing so, live a healthier life. The Campaign for Action on Salt and Health (CASH) state: 'Our bodies need a little bit of salt to survive, but the amount we eat is far more than we require.'[1]

The pedants among us argue that when it comes to the amount of salt that we *need*, it is unscientific to say we need 'a little bit' but then say we eat 'far more than we require'. Both qualifications are generalisations and the implication is that every single person is eating too much salt.

Currently the average UK resident eats an average of 8g of salt a day and the official government guidelines are 6g a day. We need somewhere between 1g and 6g. Babies will be at the lower end and athletes — who sweat more than most of us — are well above the guideline 6g or the average 8g level. Many factors are likely to influence the amount of salt different bodies require, and having a one-size-fits-all guideline doesn't work at an individual level.

Some people are larger than others. Some people sweat more than others. Some are better than others at processing salt through the kidneys. To us, there is no logic to accepting that the amounts of calories we need are variable but the amount of salt we need is fixed.

In *The Salt Fix: Why the Experts Got It All Wrong — And How Eating More Might Save Your Life*, Dr James DiNicolantonio goes into extensive detail on the research into the links between excess salt consumption and health. While we cannot necessarily endorse his central assertion — that eating more salt might save your life — it is interesting to read how research has been used to justify and support anti-salt publicity to an excessive degree.

---

1 www.actiononsalt.org.uk/salthealth/

It is commonly asserted that 75 per cent of the average person's salt allowance is found in the processed foods they eat, leaving them in control of 25 per cent of their salt intake — about 2g a day. One way to know exactly how much salt you're eating is to minimise your processed food intake and cook from scratch whenever you can, so you can control closer to 100 per cent of your daily salt intake.

What happens when we don't have enough salt?

What happens when we have too much salt is well publicised. But what happens when we don't have enough?

One scientific analysis by Dr Simon Galloway states that, 'Sodium deficiency is associated with several common modern lifestyle ailments like weakness, fatigue, depression, apathy, emotional instability, inadequate stomach acid, and memory impairment … Symptoms include nausea, vomiting, muscle cramps, loss of balance, fainting, fatigue, lethargy, depression, lack of concentration, memory impairment and forgetfulness, irritability, confusion, disorientation, emotional instability, social withdrawal, weight loss and anorexia, headache, illusions, stupor or even coma.'[2]

Dr Galloway goes on to say that these symptoms are often treated as illnesses and the drugs prescribed do not address the underlying cause. He says, 'The condition responds well to dietary modification and salt replacement to normal sodium levels.'

We need salt for life and we cannot store it, so it must be acquired from the diet.

2 *The Diagnosis and Treatment of Common Functional Illnesses: A Guide for Doctors, Practitioners and Scientists* by Simon Galloway, p335

As we've already mentioned, not all salts are created equal. There are two big differences that almost always apply. The first is that sea salt contains a variety of trace elements as well as sodium, including calcium, potassium and magnesium. All are needed by the human body. Table salt does not contain these three elements unless they are added after manufacture. This alone is a good argument for always using sea salt and not necessarily taking supplements in the form of pills or powders. Dairy, fresh fruit and vegetables will also contain these key minerals — although as we'll discover, some modern farming methods means the nutritional value has declined in recent years.

The second big difference between premium sea salts and table salts is what's added to the latter to make them 'free-flowing'. This allows salt to flow out of the saltcellar, rather than getting clogged up with moisture. And from a food manufacturer's perspective, it's easier to handle at the drying and packing stage if the granules don't form clumps. It also allows people like crisp manufacturers to add very exact amounts of salt to their products.

Table salt ingredients may list Sodium Hexacyanoferrate II (E535) or Calcium Silicate (E552) as the most common flow enhancers. We don't want to frighten anyone but the latter's other uses include insulation, fire proofing and as an ingredient in cement. These 'anticaking agents' work in two ways. Either every granule is coated with the chemical to make them water repellent, or the additive makes every granule absorb excess moisture. Neither seem desirable or necessary for good food.

Some salts contain 'natural' anticaking agents like calcium carbonate or magnesium carbonate but arguably even these can be superfluous. Carefully made natural sea salt always wants to return to a liquid state in the presence of moisture and so it follows that it's easier for your body to excrete.

Major trace elements and health

There are plenty of other good minerals in sea salt. All are absolutely essential to our health and well-being with many symptoms showing in those whose diet is deficient in them. All deficiencies eventually lead to functional illnesses — those where modern medication isn't needed, just the right healthy diet. We have already referred to Dr Simon Galloway's analysis of sodium deficiency. The same handbook has extensive references to deficiencies in calcium, potassium and magnesium. These all have key parts to play in making us literally what we are and, along with water, are the major make-up of the human body.

Declining levels of nutrients in soil and fruit and vegetables

Fresh fruit and veg also contain the minerals we need to function. However, while researching how to make sea salt we came across statistics showing the declining levels of nutrients in the vegetables we eat. This could be because farmers focus on the primary fertilisers of nitrogen, phosphorus and potassium as they are directly linked to increasing volume of crops. But secondary fertilisers are still essential.

When research was conducted by independent researcher Anne-Marie Mayer in 1997, the only mineral nutrient that showed no significant difference over the

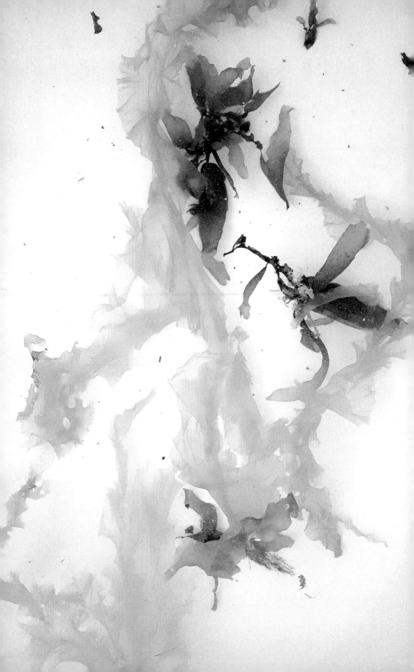

50-year period was phosphorus. This isn't surprising as phosphorus is a key constituent of commercial fertiliser but the significant decline in the others underlines the importance of obtaining them from different sources.

Evidence of the declining mineral nutrients in fruit and veg supports the hypothesis that our diet is becoming poorer. We are farming less sustainably and our soil health continues to decline. Having mineral-rich sea salt as part of our diet is a small step in the right direction for us, though we still have work to do to look after our planet.

Thalassotherapy

This is the general term used to cover the well-being benefits of using sea-related materials for purposes other than eating. An alternative way to get essential minerals into our bodies is by absorption through the skin, and people have been enjoying the benefits of bathing in magnesium-rich water for centuries.

Thalassotherapy can also include: saline nasal sprays for congestion relief, gargling with saltwater to help a sore throat, reducing inflammation and mucus in the lungs, improving respiratory conditions such as asthma and allergies, and even sitting in a salt cave to improve mood and health. All promote general well-being and many claim specific health benefits as a result. This isn't the place to examine every claim in detail but we have conducted some of our own research on nasal sprays to clean and invigorate the nose. Though initially it doesn't seem a natural pairing for gourmet sea salt sales, we are fascinated by what else our clean seawater can offer us.

Our nasal passages are like filters, yet unlike a machine whose filters are periodically cleaned, most of us don't do anything more than blow our noses. We are working with an ear, nose and throat surgeon and a PhD student at Bangor University to look at how the right concentration of seawater can provide real congestion relief.

If we are 'bunged up' our food is relatively flavourless. One simple way to demonstrate this is to peel and cut up a raw potato and a raw apple into cubes. Close your eyes and get someone to feed you random chunks; how easy is it to identify which is which? (Spoiler alert: not at all.) Indeed, 80 per cent of our sense of taste comes from our sense of smell; so it follows that we should keep our noses as clean and clear as possible. Europeans, and North Americans especially, use a brine nasal wash routinely as part of their cleansing rituals. It's less well known in Britain but early research indicates its efficacy, and it may become as much part of our daily lives as cleaning our teeth.

———————

Salt consumption is a complex and controversial subject. We wanted this chapter to shed some light on the benefits of this ingredient, as well as explore the dangers. There is, of course, overwhelming evidence that too much salt is medically bad for you, but unlike sugar, we physically need it to survive. There is also evidence to suggest that the trace elements found in sea salts are key to our health — and plenty to suggest that the sea has more to offer us than a seasoning for our chips.

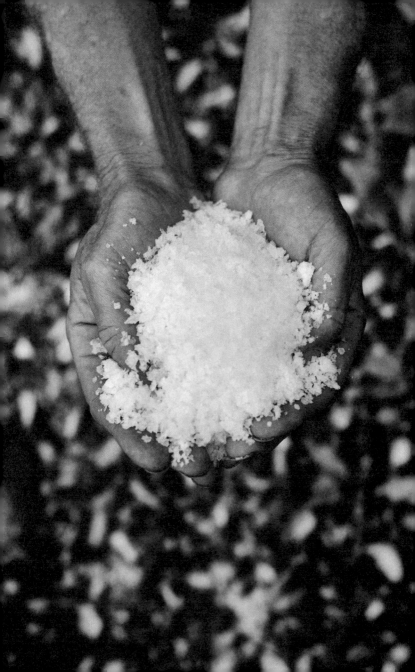

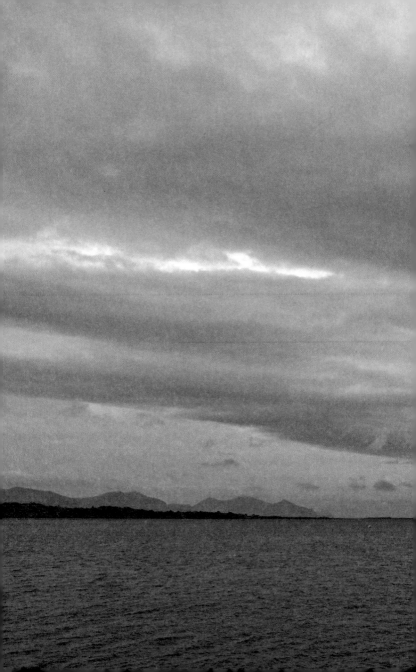

Afterword

Forget not the salt

—

Elizabeth de Grey, Countess of Kent,
A True Gentlewoman's Delight, 1688

Throughout this book we have talked about balance. The balance of getting the seasoning right: that sweet spot between too much and not enough salt, to enhance but not drown out flavour. The balance of our internal health: we need salt for our bodies to work properly but too much can make us gravely ill. And the balance and perspective that the sea brings us when we are near it.

There is no other ingredient quite like salt.

It has been revered throughout history. Struggles over who has controlled it have been the catalyst of uprisings and changes of rule. Through the centuries, it has cleansed and purified us physically and spiritually, both when we are alive and after we die.

On a personal level, the sea and the salt it contains has been the constant to our lives on Anglesey for more than 40 years. Like many people, we love living by the coast. Our daily walk along the water's edge with our two dogs gives us time to think and breathe as we enjoy the smell, sound and occasional spray of the waves. And if we're in the mood, sea bathing can be stimulating or soothing, depending on the season and the ocean. But it always makes us feel better. Our skin is softer, our hair curlier and our bodies are more relaxed.

As a rich source of sodium, magnesium, calcium and potassium, elements that we cannot live without, the health of the sea is as important for us as the health of the land. The two are irrevocably linked through the soil, and ultimately the crops and foods we eat. We think there is something deep and primeval about appreciating our natural resources and what they can offer us. So we monitor the sea's health every day, visually checking, taking a sample to test its salinity and analysing for different minerals.

Salt literally runs through our veins. It's the reason we get up in the morning, it's what we put in a warm bath before we go to bed at night.

We hope you have enjoyed this sprinkle of recollections, recipes and knowledge and that it encourages you to look again at this humblest of basic ingredients. May it also encourage you to change how you use this seasoning. Most of all, we hope that you rediscover its magical qualities for yourself.

Glossary

Black salt

Kala namak or *bire noon* is a type of rock salt, a salty and pungent-smelling condiment used in South Asia. The condiment is made of sodium chloride with several other components lending the salt its colour and smell. The smell is mainly due to added sulphur. Found mostly in the Himalayas.

Brine

Technically, this is a midway stage between seawater and sea salt. Though in cooking terms, brine just refers to a salty water of any percentage. In sea-salt-making, the strength of brine varies between 10 and 20 per cent sodium chloride depending on the stage in the evaporation.

Brining

This is the submerging of (usually) a piece of meat or poultry in a bath of salted, spiced water (technically, it's a type of curing, see below). The salt and water within the meat cells balance with the salt and water in the surrounding saltwater, which results in a higher concentration of salt and water in the meat, making it moist and delicious.

Curing

The act of preserving or flavouring meat or fish, by smoking, dehydrating or salting it.

Fine salt

Exactly what it sounds like — this usually refers to the size of the salt granules. It can be sea or rock salt.

Flake / flaked / flaky salt
Sea salt that has been evaporated slowly so that crystals form on the surface. Under a magnifying glass these will be seen to be inverted small square pyramids which form around a nucleus and then get bigger until surface tension is overcome.

Fleur de sel
Literally 'flower of the sea', this salt is French in origin and is only made in very still conditions in the South or West of France. A fine surface layer of chalk flecks appears and is largely discarded, before salt crystals form and are harvested by hand with a net. The genuine process is rare and labour intensive. Some palates detect that *fleur de sel* is 'sweeter' than sea salt.

Ground salt
Salt that goes through a grinding mill to give it a flour-like texture. Most often used in the food industry to apply a continuous stream to foods like crisps.

Iodised salt
This is table salt with added iodine. Originally it was created to prevent goitres, abnormal enlargements of the thyroid gland. In some countries, it is added by law. The iodine may give a slightly metallic taint or flavour.

Kosher salt
Traditionally, this is a coarse-grained salt used in koshering, the Jewish process where blood is removed from meat. More common in North America than Britain, famous kosher brands are Morton's or Diamond Crystal. To add a layer of confusion, actually any salt can be kosher if the process has been inspected by a rabbi (Halen Môn is kosher).

Osmosis

A process by which molecules pass through a semipermeable membrane from a less concentrated solution into a more concentrated one. Salt triggers osmosis by attracting the water and causing it to move toward it.

Pink salt

Commonly known as Himalayan salt, but not actually from the Himalayas! It is mostly sourced from the Khewra Salt Mine in Pakistan, about 300 miles to the west of the Himalayan Mountain Range. The pinkness comes from 1 per cent potassium minerals formed when shallow inland seas evaporated 1,200 million years ago. No known scientific proof exists of any health benefits of 'Himalayan' salt over other salts.

Rock salt

Sea salt that's several million years old that has dried out and been compressed into 'rock'. Commonly mined or dissolved in a little water before being chemically stripped of trace elements and made into table salt.

Salt

Usually refers to sodium chloride, which is a compound with the chemical formula NaCl. Chlorine on its own is a toxic gas. Sodium is used, amongst other things, to fuel streetlights, giving them their orange hue. Together these elements form a strong bond and give us the seasoning.

Confusingly, the word 'salts' can also refer to compounds other than sodium chloride. For example, saltpetre (sodium nitrite) and natron. Sea salt contains 90–95% sodium chloride and the balance is made up of other 'salts' such as magnesium chloride and potassium chloride, sulphates, trace elements and moisture.

Sea salt
The salt made from evaporating seawater. Sea salt retains many valuable trace elements if made traditionally.

Seawater
Typically raw seawater has 3.5 per cent salt content.

Sel gris
Literally 'grey salt', this is a coarse granular sea salt popularised by the French. Coarser than *fleur de sel* and characterised by being very moist. The colour comes from the salt being allowed to come into contact with the bottom of the salt pan (usually a shallow wide trench on the shore line) before being raked into a pile.

Table salt
Still the most commonly used salt. Usually made in bulk in a vacuum evaporator system. There are little other essential minerals in table salt, as opposed to in sea salt, which retains a lot of other trace minerals which our bodies need. It often has an anticaking agent added too, to stop clumping. (*See also* rock salt.)

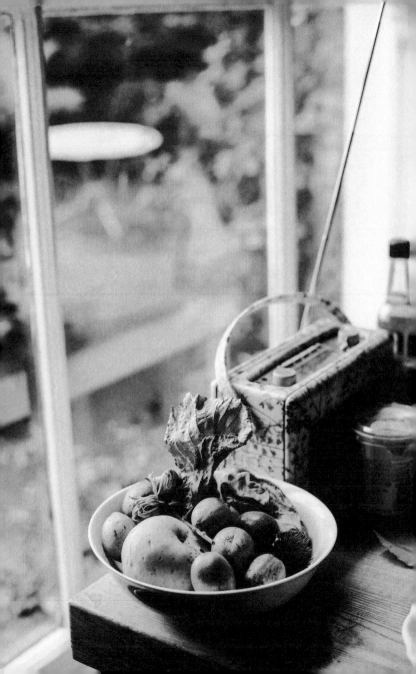

Resources

Read

Salt: A World History by Mark Kurlansky

Salted: A Manifesto on the World's Most Essential Mineral, with Recipes by Mark Bitterman

It Must've Been Something I Ate by Jeffrey Steingarten

The Diagnosis and Treatment of Common Functional Illnesses by Simon Galloway

The SAS Survival Handbook by John 'Lofty' Wiseman Essentials: Facing Disaster: Water and Salt

The Salt Fix: Why The Experts Got It All Wrong and How Eating More Might Save Your Life by Dr James DiNicolantonio

Spices, Salt and Aromatics in the English Kitchen by Elizabeth David

Watch

Samin Nosrat's Netflix series, *Salt Fat Acid Heat*

Alison and David Lea-Wilson, 'Why we should value true eccentricity', *thedolectures.com*

Visit

The beach in front of Halen Môn in Brynsiencyn — the place that started it all

Wieliczka Salt Mine in Krakow — for a tour like no other

ActiononSalt.org.uk

Listen

Radio 4's The Food Programme — episode on Salt, via iPlayer

Eat

Fran's Caramels, Seattle: *frans.com*

Stone Barns — ingredient-led cooking in New York

'O ver restaurant — saltwater cooking in London

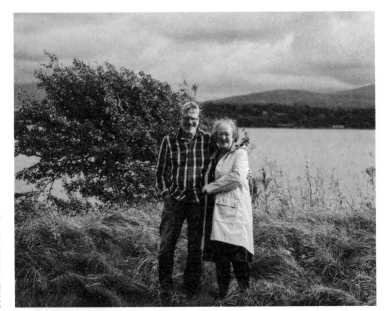

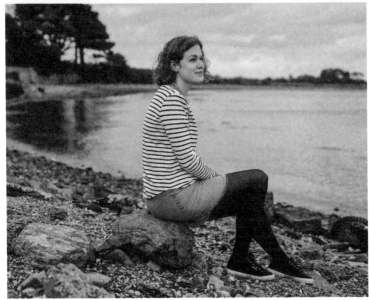

About the authors

Alison and David Lea-Wilson started Halen Môn, the Anglesey Sea Salt company, in 1997. They have always made a living from the sea — first as fishmongers, then aquarium owners — and been fascinated by the process of making sea salt.

In 2017, Halen Môn won the Queen's Award for Sustainability, and in 2019, Alison and David were awarded MBEs for their services to business.

Their daughter, Jess, is a writer and designer who has worked in the food industry her whole working life. She loves talking about vegetarian food: making it, writing about it, but most of all, eating it.

Thanks

Thank you to our wonderful editor Miranda for taking on three authors at once, for all your expertise and perhaps most of all, for your patience! And to Imogen, Wilf, Fiona — thank you for all of the parts you have played in bringing this book to life. Anna Shepherd — thank you for everything. Not sure if we are more grateful for your friendship or for your absolutely delicious recipes. Shane Lyons, thank you for being an integral part of *Do Sea Salt*. We are so glad we walked into Distilled NY, it changed our lives for the better. Liz and Max — your photographs do the incredible island that we call home justice, and that is a real achievement. Matt Russell — your images are simply beautiful, thank you. Eamon Fullalove — in many ways, the seed for this book started with you. Thank you. John Mitchinson, thank you for believing in our book from the very beginning. We appreciate your faith in us, even if the first incarnation didn't go according to plan! Anna Jones — thank you for all the support you have shown our company and our family. Life is more delicious because of you and Jess feels exceptionally lucky to work with you. Brandt and Micah — becoming an ingredient in Green + Black's chocolate has been one of many highlights in our company history. Thank you for using our products and sharing your expertise in these pages.

To all the staff at Halen Môn, thank you for making it what it is today. Thank you especially to Nicki, for your unfailing support for well over a decade. Sam, we are so excited for what is to come at Halen Môn. Thank you for your careful testing. Thank you to the chemistry department of Bangor University, which has been an incredible asset to us over the years. Richard — thank you for putting your Blue Peter hat back on and helping us make sea salt at home again!

Special thanks to the Do Lectures: we have found so much inspiration in your community. Your encouragement has helped fuel our constant innovation and set our sights ever higher.

Finally, to all of our family: thank you, thank you, thank you. Running a family business is an all-encompassing affair, with many highs and lows. Thank you for living and breathing sea salt. Thank you especially to Hamish, Jake and Margaret. (Thanks to Josie too for putting up with a family who discusses what to have for lunch before breakfast is finished!) Reg, Joy, Ian — we wish you could have seen this book.

Index

Books in the series

Also available

Book Co

Available in print, digital and audio formats from booksellers or via our website: **thedobook.co**

To hear about events and forthcoming titles, you can find us on social media **@dobookco**, or subscribe to our newsletter